MW01047810

RECENT TCM RESEARCH
FROM CHINA

RECENT TCM
RESEARCH
FROM CHINA

1991-1994

translated by

Bob Flaws
and
Charles Chace

BLUE POPPY PRESS

Published by:

BLUE POPPY PRESS
1775 LINDEN AVE.
BOULDER, CO 80304

FIRST EDITION, MAY 1994

ISBN 0-936185-56-2, LC# 94-70761

COPYRIGHT 1994 © BLUE POPPY PRESS

The information in this book is given in good faith. However, the translators and the publisher cannot be held responsible for any error or omission. Nor can they be held in any way responsible for treatment given on the basis of information contained in this book. The publisher make this information available to English language readers for scholarly and research purposes only.

The publishers do not advocate nor endorse self-medication by laypersons. Chinese medicine is a professional medicine. Laypersons interested in availing themselves of the treatments described in this book should seek out a qualified professional practitioner of Chinese medicine.

Printed at Westview Press, Boulder, CO on acid free, recycled paper.
Cover printed at C & M Press, Thornton, CO.

COMP Designation: Functionally translated abstracts using a standard technical terminology

10 9 8 7 6 5 4 3 2

Preface

This book is a collection of functionally translated abstracts from recent Chinese medical journals. They are functionally translated in that they have not been translated word for word. Rather, we have translated only what we felt was the most important, clinically useful information in each article. Nonetheless, the translators based their terminology on Nigel Wiseman & Ken Boss' *Glossary of Chinese Medical Terms and Acupuncture Points*.

The book is divided into a number of sections, similar to many modern Chinese TCM journals. There are sections on *nei ke*, internal medicine; *fu ke*, gynecology; *er ke*, pediatrics; *pi fu ke*, dermatology; *nan ke*, urology & male sexual dysfunction; *shang gu ke*, traumatology & orthopedics; and *zhen jiu tui na*, acupuncture/moxibustion & medical massage. Under each of these chapter headings, one will find a number of diseases, and under these diseases, one will find one or more articles or research reports. The reader should note, however, that under acupuncture/moxibustion & *tui na*, there are articles on *nei ke, fu ke, er ke, nan ke,* and *pi fu ke*.

This underscores the fact that in modern China, acupuncture and moxibustion are seen as a somewhat separate, self-contained modality. In addition, the names of many of the journals we have translated these articles from include the words *zhong yi yao. Zhong* means Chinese, *yi* means medicine, and *yao* means herbs or medicinals. *Yi yao* can be read simply as a compound term meaning medicine. However, even still, it points up the fact that herbal medicine is the main modality in modern Chinese medicine. Unless the journal is specifically an acupuncture/moxibustion journal, acupuncture/-moxibustion and *tui na* usually comprise only 1/10 or less of any Chinese TCM journal's articles.

Many of these articles are reports on clinical audits. Typically, Chinese TCM practitioners do not do double-blinded, placebo-controlled research. A clinical audit is where one goes back through their records and tallies the results of every patient with a certain disease who was given the same treatment. Such clinical audits can, therefore, be done in retrospect. After having seen a number of cases of a particular disease, one simply see how many were cured, how many were markedly improved, and how many got no result with a certain treatment and in what time span. Basically, this type of research results in uncontrolled amelioration rates.

In such clinical audits, there is no attempt to insure that the patients seen are a statistically representative cross-section of either the general population or the population of sufferers with that disease. Nor is there any attempt to identify or rule out placebo effect. The bottom line is simply how many patients a practitioner or group of practitioners were able to treat effectively with a certain protocol. As the reader will see, most of the amelioration rates given typically total in the 90% range. From a very practical point of view, this is really all a clinician needs to know. We need to know if a given treatment benefits a majority of the patients who receive it and that there are no, or minimal side effects.

Because modern Western medicine and its allies, insurance and pharmaceutical companies, do clinical audits for most diseases, it should be possible to compare the costs and effectiveness of the treatments in this book with modern Western medicine's standard of care for the same diseases. Therefore, we are publishing this book as a resource both for clinicians in their day to day practice and also for those who wish to fight for the licensing of acupuncture and Chinese medicine and its reimbursement by third party payers, such as insurance companies, Medicaid, Medicare, and Worker's Compensation.

Further, it is hoped that this book may serve as the source of research protocols to be done by Western practitioners and as a source of treatment protocols for diseases not covered in English language TCM textbooks. For instance, the protocol for the treatment of oral aphthae (thrush) might be adopted for research among HIV patients with fluconazole-resistant patients. Or one of the herpes zoster protocols might be adopted for HIV herpes zoster sufferers who cannot afford Acyclovir. In addition, the clinician will find herein, treatments for a number of diseases and conditions with which their patients may present but which do not appear in *Chinese Acupuncture & Moxibustion* and other such existing English language texts. For instance, the practitioner will find effective treatments for hypersensitive and chronically inflamed lips, anal itching, post-abortion bleeding, menstrual pneumothorax, Tourette's Syndrome, and other often overlooked but very real human health dilemmas.

Other of the articles are more theoretical in nature. Rather than discussing the research outcomes of a particular protocol, the author may discuss some over-looked point in the practice of TCM. Usually these essays are supported by case histories. They often can clarify some knotty problem in either diagnosis or treatment. Personally, I find reading these Chinese journal articles a gold mine of information, and having once delved into this treasure trove, I do not know how I could go back to practicing in ignorance of them.

Over the last decade or more, Blue Poppy Press has tried to publish representatives of every major genre of Chinese medical literature. We have published the Great Masters Series, a collection of translations of preeminent Chinese medical classics, numerous textbooks on various clinical specialties, several collections of medical essays, and one case history compilation. However, the Chinese journal literature is largely unknown to Western practitioners who cannot read medical Chinese. Every one to two months, approximately 40 such journals are published in the People's Republic of China. These are published by provincial TCM presses, by TCM colleges, by TCM research associations, by acupuncture/moxibustion associations, and by *qi gong* associations. Each journal typically contains several dozen articles on a wide variety of subjects. As mentioned above, most of this material is on internal or so-called herbal medicine, but it does include acupuncture/moxibustion, *tui na, qi gong,* Chinese dietary therapy, and longevity practices.

Textbooks, by their nature, only give a very cursory and theoretical overview to the practice of Chinese medicine. Although they are indispensable to students, they leave a lot unsaid. In Asia, it is assumed one's clinical mentors will fill in these gaps. However, here in the West, we have yet to develop a large cadre of senior Western practitioners who can provide knowledgeable and authoritative clinical guidance to neophytes. Most textbooks simply list treatment protocols underneath diseases and patterns, but in clinical practice, these may only work a percentage of the time. It is journal articles such as contained herein which give the record of the actual implementation of specific treatment protocols and their outcomes. As such, we Westerners need access to this kind of literature even more than our Asian counterparts. At least one well known American TCM practitioner has pointed out that those Western practitioners who cannot read modern medical Chinese are falling behind our Asian peers by several hundred articles per month.

Hopefully, the range and value of the material contained in this book will encourage students and practitioners to begin trying to read modern medical Chinese. In addition, perhaps this book will also prompt Western acupuncture and Oriental medical schools to require a reading knowledge of Chinese or some other Asian language of every single student. As I have demonstrated to numerous students over the years, one can begin reading modern Chinese TCM journal articles with the help of dictionaries and glossaries within three months. Slowly and laboriously, granted, but with time, one will pick up speed and need to look up fewer and fewer words. Charles Chace studied Chinese language while a student at the New England School of Acupuncture and has done extensive tutorial work. Nevertheless, we are both largely self-taught. If we have been able to translate these abstracts into English, it is primarily due to interest coupled with perseverance.

The reader will note some minor differences in terminology between the two translators. Also, each translator has their own style of writing English. Hopefully these differences will show that different people can use the same standard TCM glossary and yet produce their own idiosyncratic prose. In other words, the use of such a standard glossary does not have to result in the complete homogenization of the English language TCM literature.

We have not translated the word *ji* (剂). Literally, this word means formula or prescription. However, as used in modern Chinese TCM textbooks and journal articles, it refers to the number of individual packets of medicine prescribed or used. Each packet contains one whole formula. Therefore, in Chinese, one can speak of the number of formulas prescribed or taken. In this context, this word is thus synonymous with *bao* or packet.

The translator of each article is identified by their initials appearing directly after the page number in the bibliographic information following the title and author's name. BF stands for Bob Flaws and CC stands for Charles Chace.

Bob Flaws
February 20, 1994

Contents

Nan Ke/Urology & Male Sexual Dysfunction

Er Ke/Pediatrics

Pi Fu Ke/Dermatology

Shang Gu Ke/Traumatology & Orthopedics

Zhen Jiu Tui Na/Acupuncture/Moxibustion & Medical Massage

Acupuncture

Moxibustion

Tui Na

Miscellaneous Articles _____

Nei Ke
Internal Medicine _____

Oral Thrush

"100 Cases of Recurrent Oral Aphthae (*i.e.*, Thrush) Treated by *Kou Kui Ting* (Mouth Ulcer Stopper)" by He Bo & Jin Cui-yi, *Hu Bei Zhong Yi Za Zhi (The Hubei Journal of Traditional Chinese Medicine)*, #5, 1993, p. 23; BF

This clinical audit reports on the treatment of 100 cases of recurrent oral thrush with *Kou Kui Ting* from the beginning of 1987 to the end of 1992. Besides the recurrent thrush, accompanying symptoms included insomnia, excessive dreams, lack of strength, poor appetite, loose stools, nose and throat pain, nervous tension, emotional instability, early or late menstruation, and a tendency to recurrent flus. Among the 100 cases, 34 were men and 66 were women. Twenty cases were between 14-20 years of age, and 80 were between 21-50. The shortest course of disease was 1 year and the longest 10 years. Within any 1-2 week period, 10 cases experienced 1 flare-up. Within any 2-3 week period, 20 cases experienced a flare-up. Within any 3-4 week period, 31 cases experienced a flare-up. While 25 cases experienced flare-ups during indeterminate periods and 14 cases experienced oral aphthae continuously.

The treatment method consisted of taking 15g each of: Radix Isatidis Seu Baphicacanthi (*Ban Lang Gen*), Radix Bupleuri (*Chai Hu*), Radix Astragali Membranacei (*Huang Qi*), and Fructificatio Tremellae (*Yin Er*). These were decocted and processed, turning them into a 200% water preparation. Each day, 3 doses of 30ml each were given, and 4-6 weeks comprised 1 course of treatment.

Results were defined as follows: Cure consisted of disappearance of the oral aphthae with 1 course of treatment and no recurrence within 1 year. Partial results consisted of 2-3 recurrences after 2-3 courses of treatment with a general lessening of the condition's severity and shortening of its course. While no results meant that, after 2-3 courses of treatment, the patient continued to have recurrences each month. Based on these definitions, 82 cases were cured, 16 received some results, and 2 cases experienced no results.

According to He and Jin's discussion, within this formula, Isatis clears heat and resolves toxins, disinhibits the throat and disperses swelling. Bupleurum courses the liver and resolves depression thus relaxing one's emotions. Therefore, there is no mechanism for transformative heat from internal accumulation. Astragalus supplements the center and boosts the qi so that the spleen's transportation is strengthened, the clear yang is up-borne, and vacuity fire automatically restrained. Tremella enriches yin, nourishes the stomach, and generates fluids. As a whole, this formula is neither excessively cold or warm. It clears without damaging yin, while it supplements without aiding evils.

Mouth & Tongue Dryness

"The Pattern Discrimination Treatment of 32 Cases of Mouth & Tongue Dryness Condition" by Hu Yong, Hu Yan, & Shang Zu-bo, *Ji Lin Zhong Yi Yao (Jilin Traditional Chinese Medicine & Medicinals)*, #5, 1993, p. 26; BF

This brief report describes the treatment of 32 cases of mouth and tongue dryness condition. In this study, 9 patients were men and 23 were women. The youngest was 35 years old and the oldest was 69. All the patients had a dry mouth with diminished saliva or a pasty feeling mouth. Half the cases had a scorching heat in their mouths with a coarse, rough feeling. Some had occasional ulcers in their throats inhibiting their swallowing. Taste was reduced, the lips were chapped, the corners of the mouth were chapped, and the tongue was dry and red colored.

Pattern discrimination & treatment:

1. Internal dryness damages fluids. In order to moisten dryness and protect fluids, *Xi Jiao Di Huang Tang Jia Jian* (Rhinoceros Horn & Rehmannia Decoction with Additions & Subtractions) was administered.

2. Kidney yin insufficiency. In order to enrich yin and clear heat, engender fluids and stop thirst, *Zhi Bai Di Huang Tang Jia Jian* (Anemarrhena & Phellodendron, Rehmannia Decoction with Additions & Subtractions) was given.

3. Qi & yin dual vacuity. In order to boost the qi and nourish yin, enrich, moisten, and engender fluids, *Sheng Mai San Jia Jian* (Engender the Pulse Powder with Additions & Subtractions) was given.

4. Spleen & stomach vacuity weakness. In order to fortify the spleen and eliminate dampness, boost the stomach and disseminate fluids, *Bu Zhong Yi Qi Tang Jia Jian* (Supplement the Center, Boost the Qi Decoction with Additions & Subtractions) was given.

5. Kidney yang insufficiency. In order to warm and supplement kidney yang, disseminate and engender fluids, *Jin Gui Shen Qi Tang Jia Jian* (Golden Cabinet Kidney Qi Decoction with Additions & Subtractions) was given.

Of the 32 cases, 16 were cured, meaning that their mouth and tongue dryness disappeared with no recurrence within 3 months. Six cases were improved, meaning that their mouth and tongue dryness basically disappeared. And 6 cases experienced no result. Two weeks constituted 1 course of treatment. One can expect results after 1 whole course of therapy. The combined amelioration rate was 81.3%.

"The Treatment of Senile Dryness Syndrome with *Zhi Bai Di Huang Tang Jia Jian* (Anemarrhena & Phellodendron Rehmannia Decoction with Additions & Subtractions)" by Zhang Lan-cao, *Ji Lin Zhong Yi Yao (Jilin Traditional Chinese Medicine & Medicinals)*, #3, 1993, p. 24; BF

Senile dryness syndrome is a commonly seen condition in clinical practice. It consists of mouth dryness even to the point of ulcers of the oral cavity, difficulty swallowing, and a hoarse voice. In addition, the stools may be dry even to the point of causing anal fissures, prolapse of the anus, and itching. Because this is a chronic disease, long-term administration of medicinals is typically required. The author has treated 24 cases of this condition with *Zhi Bai Di Huang Tang Jia Jian*. All these patients were treated as out-patients. Sixteen were men and 8 were women. The youngest was 56 years old and the oldest was 71. Fifteen had dryness of the mouth and nose, while 9 had dry stools.

The medicinals used consisted of: Rhizoma Anemarrhenae (*Zhi Mu*), 20g, Cortex Phellodendri (*Huang Bai*), 20g, prepared Radix Rehmanniae (*Shu Di*), 15g, Fructus Corni Officinalis (*Shan Zhu Yu*), 10g, Radix Dioscoreae Oppositae (*Shan Yao*), 10g, Rhizoma Alismatis (*Ze Xie*), 10g, Sclerotium Poriae Cocos (*Fu Ling*), 10g, and Cortex Radicis Moutan (*Dan Pi*), 10g. If there were dry nose and mouth, Radix Puerariae (*Ge Gen*), Radix Trichosanthis Kirlowii (*Hua Fen*), and Radix Polygoni Multiflori (*He Shou Wu*), Fructus Psoraleae Corylifoliae (*Bu Gu Zhi*), and the Three Immortals (*San Xian*) were added. If the stools were dry, Radix Polygoni Multiflori (*Shou Wu*), Fructus Psoraleae Corylifoliae (*Bu Gu Zhi*), Radix Et Rhizoma Rhei (*Da Huang*), Semen Pruni (*Yu Li Ren*), Rhizoma Polygonati Odorati (*Yu Zhu*), and Herba Dendrobii (*Shi Hu*) were added.

Of the 15 cases of dry nose and mouth, 12 or 80% were cured, 2 or 13.3% received fair improvement, and 1 got no result. Of the 9 cases of dry stools, 5 or 55.5% were cured, 3 or 33.3% received fair improvement, and 1 got no result. The average treatment consisted of 12 _ji_ of medicinals.

Allergic Rhinitis

"The Treatment of 42 Cases of Allergic Rhinitis with _Si Wu Tang Jia Wei_ (Four Materials Decoction with Added Flavors)" by Li Guang-zhen, _Ji Lin Zhong Yi Yao (Jilin Traditional Chinese Medicine & Medicinals)_, #3, 1993, p. 25; BF

Since 1985, the author has treated 42 cases of allergic rhinitis with _Si Wu Tang Jia Wei_. Of these 42, 29 were men and 13 were women. They ranged in age from a young of 19 to an old of 62 years of age. The shortest course of disease was 4 months and the longest was 10 years. Runny nose, itchy nose, and sneezing were the main symptoms. Examination revealed that the nasal mucosa were either an ashen white or purplish sooty color, the nasal shell was edematous, and the nasal cavity was producing a flowing secretion. Examination of the nasal secretions were positive for eosinophilia.

The medicinals consisted of: raw Radix Rehmanniae (_Sheng Di_), 24g, Radix Angelicae Sinensis (_Dang Gui_) and Radix Rubrus Paeoniae Lactiflorae (_Chi Shao_), 15g @, Rhizoma Ligustici Wallichii (_Chuan Xiong_), 6g, Fructus Xanthii (_Cang Er Zi_) and Flos Magnoliae (_Xin Yi_), 9g @, and Herba Pycnostelmae (_Xu Chang Jing_), 30g. If there was headache, Radix Angelicae (_Bai Zhi_) and Flos Chrysanthemi Morifolii (_Ju Hua_) were added. If there was a cold (_gan mao_), these medicinals were combined with _Yu Ping Feng San_ (Jade Windscreen Powder). One _ji_ was decocted per day with 15 days equalling 1 course of treatment. Two to 4 courses of treatment were given with a follow-up survey conducted 1 year after treatment.

Twenty-three patients were completely cured. This meant that their symptoms disappeared, their nasal mucosa and secretions returned to normal, and their nasal secretions tested negative for eosinophils. Thirteen cases got fair improvement. This meant that their symptoms were obviously reduced or partially disappeared. The number of attacks or the duration of attacks was also reduced, and their nasal secretions mostly tested negative for eosinophils. And 6 patients got no result from this treatment. This meant that there was no apparent change in their condition from before the treatment was begun. Therefore, the total amelioration rate was 85.7%.

According to TCM theory, the main disease mechanism of this disease is yin and blood insufficiency. In that case, constructive and defensive are empty and sparse and the exterior defensive fails to secure. This then allows for external invasion of wind cold, and this results in the portal of the lungs (*i.e.*, the nose) losing its disinhibition. *Si Wu Tang* enriches yin and nourishes blood, moves the qi and harmonizes the constructive, thus supporting the righteous. As the saying goes, "When the blood is harmonious (or harmonized), wind is automatically extinguished." Xanthium, Flos Magnoliae, and Pycnostelma diffuse the lungs, open the portals, and, therefore, dispel evils. When evils are dispelled, the righteous is at ease. With the righteous returned and evils removed, the disease obtains a cure.

Wheezing & Asthma

"Fu Yuan Huo Xue Tang Jia Jian (Revive Health by Invigorating the Blood Decoction) in the Treatment of Wheezing & Asthma" by Ru Xiao-hua, *Shang Hai Zhong Yi Yao Za*

Zhi (The Shanghai Journal of Traditional Chinese Medicine & Medicinals), #3, 1992, p. 36; CC

Fu Yuan Huo Xue Tang quickens the blood and eliminates stasis, courses the liver and unblocks the connecting vessels, and is often used in external medicine. The author has used _Fu Wan Huo Xue Tang_ with modifications in the treatment wheezing and asthma to good effect. Wheezing and asthma are most often due to inhibition of the qi dynamic with chronic depression transforming into fire. This fiery qi scorches the fluids producing phlegm. This, in turn, further obstructs the qi dynamic. Once the qi becomes chronically stagnant this results in (blood) stasis.

The formula consists of: Radix Bupleuri (_Radix Bupleuri_), 6-9g, Radix Angelicae Sinensis (_Dang Gui_), 9g, Semen Pruni Persicae (_Tao Ren_), 6-9g, Flos Carthami Tinctorii (_Hong Hua_), 5g, Radix Et Rhizoma Rhei (_Da Huang_), 6-9g, Radix Glycyrrhizae (_Gan Cao_), 5g, Radix Trichosanthis Kirlowii (_Tian Hua Fen_), 6-9g, Lumbricus (_Di Long_), 18g, Herba Ephedrae (_Ma Huang_), 9g, Radix Albus Paeoniae Lactiflorae (_Bai Shao_), 9-12g, Fructus Citri Seu Ponciri (_Zhi Ke_), 6-9g, and Fructus Xanthii (_Cang Er Zi_), 9g.

If the phlegm is thick and yellow and there is thoracic oppression, then add Fructus Trichosanthis Kirlowii (_Gua Lou_), 12g, Radix Scutellariae Baicalensis (_Huang Qin_), 9-12g, and Herba Houttuyniae Cordatae (_Yu Xing Cao_), 9-12g. If there is simultaneous vacuity of spleen and kidney yang, then add Radix Praeparatus Aconiti Carmichaeli (_Fu Zi_), 6-9g, Radix Codonopsis Pilosulae (_Dang Shen_), 9g, and Rhizoma Atractylodis Macrocephalae (_Bai Zhu_), 9-12g. For frequent wheezing and asthma, add Radix Panacis Cinquefolii (_Xi Yang Shen_) or Radix Rubrus Panacis Ginseng (_Hong Shen_), 6-9g and Gecko (_Ge Jie_), 1 pair.

In this prescription, Bupleurum, Peony, and Fructus Citri Seu Ponciri resolve depression and rectify the qi. *Dang Gui*, Persica, Carthamus, and Rhubarb quicken the blood, circulate the qi, and scatter stasis. Trichosanthes "clears vexation from the chest and stomach allowing the dirty heat to be eliminated." Lumbricus and Ephedra combine to diffuse the lung qi, disperse inflammation, and level asthma. Xanthium eliminates wind and diffuses the portals. This function is enhanced when combined with Lumbricus. The entire prescription quickens the blood and circulates stasis, rectifies the qi, transforms stagnation, and levels asthma.

The above prescription was used to treat 7 cases of wheezing and asthma ranging from 52-70 years of age. The duration of the illness ranged from 5-10 years. Chest x-rays revealed evidence of bronchial swelling. In general, the asthma was controlled after administration of from 5-10 *ji*.

"How are the Principles of Diffusing the Qi, Downbearing the Qi, Normalizing the Qi, Boosting the Qi, and Absorbing the Qi to be Understood and Used Within the Context of Wheezing?" by Shen Qing-fa, *Zhong Yi Za Zhi (The Journal of Traditional Chinese Medicine)*, #8, 1992, p. 55; CC

The primary symptoms of wheezing are its recurrent nature, the presence of a wheezing sound in the throat, shortened and rapid distressed respiration, and, in extreme cases, dyspneic breathing with an incapacity to lie down. Phlegm is a part of this pathology. The location of the disease is in the lungs, but, in long-standing cases, there may be injury to the spleen and kidneys as well. The disease transformation is at the level of the qi, and the illness may change from a repletion to a vacuity pattern. It is sometimes due to deep-lying internal phlegm precipitating a contraction of a pathogen. For instance, the section "Wheezing & Asthma" in the text, _Zheng Zhi Hui Bu (Supplemental Collection of Pattern Treatments)_ states,

> (Wheezing) is due to internal obstruction of the qi, an externally ill-timed [pathogenic] contraction, and the presence of sticky, consolidated phlegm in the chest. These three factors combine with one another to obstruct the airways and produce wheezing.

When the symptoms are not apparent, the qi and yin are gradually becoming vacuous, and the lung spleen, and kidney viscera are gradually becoming depleted. If the lung is vacuous, it is unable to govern the qi. Thus depurative downbearing has no influence, the qi is not transformed into fluid, and turbid phlegm accumulates internally. This then results in a gradual lack of security of the defensive qi on the exterior.

A vacuity of the spleen causes a failure of the transformation of water and grain qi, resulting in an accumulation of dampness that generates phlegm. This phlegm and dampness ascend and are stored within the lungs.

A vacuity of the kidney depletes the essence qi, causing a loss of assimilation and absorption. One may then observe the pattern of yang vacuity with the floating of water to produce phlegm or the pattern of yin vacuity with vacuity fire scorching the fluids to produce phlegm, both of which ascend and attack the lungs.

When wheezing does occur, pathogenic repletion is primary and treatment via depurating the lung qi, downbearing the lung qi, and normalizing the accumulation of qi is suggested. When wheezing is not apparent, vacuity of the righteous qi is primary and treatment via boosting the lung qi, supplementing the spleen qi, and assimilating insufficiency of qi is suggested. The specific utilization of these principles is described below.

Diffusion of the qi (*xuan qi*): This principle is used in phlegm rheum lying deeply within the lungs that has developed upon contact with cold. In this pattern, the following symptoms are commonly seen: asthmatic qi, fullness in the chest, a wheezing sound in the chest, a cold body, aversion to chill, cough with thin, scanty phlegm, no thirst or a desire for warm drinks, a white, slimy tongue coating, and a pulse that is wiry and replete or wiry and tense. *She Gan Ma Huang Tang* (Belamcanda & Ephedra Decoction) is selected to diffuse the lung qi, disperse cold, and transform phlegm. This prescription utilizes Rhizoma Belamcandae (*She Gan*) and Herba Ephedrae (*Ma Huang*) as the primary medicinals to diffuse the lung and level asthma on the outside. Fresh Rhizoma Zingiberis (*Sheng Jiang*) and Radix Paeoniae Lactiflorae (*Shao Yao*) are combined along with Herba Cum Radice Asari Sieboldi (*Xi Xin*) and Fructus Schizandrae Chinensis (*Wu Wei Zi*) as assistants (and envoys) to disperse cold phlegm and eliminate the phlegmatic noises and cough asthmatic counterflow. Based on the author's experience, the addition of Semen Plantaginis (*Che Qian Zi*) enhances the therapeutic effect.

Downbearing the qi (*jiang qi*): This principle is used in lung heat obstructing the lungs where the lungs have lost their function of depurative downbearing. In this pattern, the following symptoms are commonly seen: elevated chest and lateral costal distension, dyspnea and rough respiration, a howling phlegmatic sound, a reddened face and perspiration, spitting up of thick, sticky phlegm, thirst and desire for fluids, a red tongue with a slimy, yellow coating, and a slippery, rapid pulse. *Ding Chuan Tang* (Calm Wheezing Decoction) is selected to downbear the lung qi, drain heat, and transform phlegm. This prescription contains Semen Gingkonis Bilobae (*Bai Guo*) which settles asthmatic expectoration and is combined with Fructus Perillae Frutescentis (*Su Zi*) which downbears phlegmatic qi. Radix Scutellariae Baicalensis (*Huang Qin*) combined with Rhizoma Pinelliae Ternatae (*Ban Xia*) and Cortex Radicis Mori (*Sang Bai Pi*) assist Flos Tussilaginis Farfarae (*Kuan Dong Hua*. In each pair,) a cold and a warming medicinal are used together to facilitate the drainage of heat and the downbearing of counterflow. In the author's experience, the addition of Lumbricus (*Di Long*) and Bulbus Fritillariae Cirrhosae (*Chuan Bei*) enhance the effect.

Normalizing the qi (*shun qi*): This principle is used in cases of qi vacuity with an exuberance of phlegm obstructing the lungs. In this pattern, the following symptoms may be observed: (the illness) occurs repeatedly, there is a phlegmatic sound in the throat as if one were snoring, and there are a sallow, white facial complexion, perspiration and chilled extremities, a low sounding shortness of breath, a white, greasy tongue coating, and a deep, fine, and slippery pulse. *Su Zi jiang Qi Tang* (Perilla Decoction to Downbear the Qi) normalizes obstructions in the qi. This prescription employs Fructus Perillae Frutescentis (*Su Zi*) and Rhizoma Pinellia Ternatae (*Ban Xia*) to downbear the qi and transform phlegm. Cortex Magnoliae Officinalis (*Hou Po*) and Pericarpium Citri Reticulatae (*Chen Pi*) normalize the qi and harmonize the middle. And Cortex Cinnamomi (*Rou Gui*) and Radix Angelicae Sinensis (*Dang Gui*) warm and nourish the kidney qi. The normalization of the obstruction of the lung qi is a branch treatment, while supplementation of the kidney vacuity below is a root treatment. In the author's experience, the combination of *San Zi Yang Xi Tang* (Three Seed Decoction to Nourish One's Parents) with Fluoritum (*Zi Shi Ying*) may be used in the same manner.

Boosting the qi (*yi qi*): This principle is used in cases of wheezing patterns requiring resolution measures that are also characterized by a vacuity of lung and spleen qi. The following symptoms may be observed: There is a tendency to catch colds, a low sounding shortness of breath, a weak, forceless voice, hacking up thin, white, viscous phlegm, an occasional phlegmatic sound, gastric *pi*, diminished intake, pasty stools, a pale tongue, and a fine, weak pulse. In this case, the prescription used is *Yu Ping Feng San* (Jade Wind Screen Powder) in combination with modified *Shen Ling Bai Zhu San* (Ginseng, Poria, & Atractylodes Powder).

Assimilation of the qi (*na qi*): This principle is used in wheezing patterns of a long-standing nature with kidney vacuity resulting in a failure of absorption and assimilation. The symptoms are dyspnea and rapid distressed respiration, and shortness of breath, difficulty with inhalation, a white facial complexion and cold body, low back and knee soreness and weakness, a pale, inflated tongue body, and a sunken, fine pulse. The prescription is *You Gui Wan* (Restore the Right Pills) in combination with modified *Shen Jie San* (Ginseng & Gecko Powder). The author prefers to use prepared Radix Rehmanniae (*Shu Di Huang*), Fructus Corni Officinalis (*Shan Yu Rou*), Radix Morindae (*Ba Ji Rou*), Semen Juglandis Regiae (*Hu Tao Ren*), Fructus Psoraleae Corylifoliae (*Bu Gu Zhi*), and Fluoritum (*Zi Shi Ying*) as a foundation for herbal prescription. Then, based on a discrimination of patterns, Placenta Hominis (*Zi He Che*), Lumbricus (*Di Long*), and powdered Os Sepiae Seu Sepiellae (*Hai Piao Xiao*) may be added to the prescription to ensure a therapeutic effect.

"The Treatment of Wheezing & Dyspnea With Medicated Plasters Applied to Acupoints" by Li Zhi, *Hu Nan Zhong Yi Za Zhi (The Hunan Journal of Traditional Chinese Medicine)*, #1, 1993, p. 25-7; BF

This clinical audit describes the treatment of 800 cases of wheezing and dyspnea through the application of medicated plasters on acupoints. Of the 800 patients, 560 were male and 240 were female. There were 50 cases involving patients 20 years old or less; 60 involving those 30 years old or less; 70 cases, 40 years old or less; 200 cases, 50 years old or less; and 400 cases involving patients 51 years or older. The duration of these patients' disease ranged from 110 cases, 5 years or less; 120 cases, 10 years or less; 200 cases, 15 years or less; and 375 cases, 15 years or more. Further, 275 cases were categorized as light, 400 as moderate, and 125 as severe. In addition, 610 cases were diagnosed as cold pattern dyspnea, 150 as hot pattern dyspnea, and 40 cases fell into the so-called other category.

Depending upon the type of wheezing and dyspnea, any of three different _gao_ or pastes were applied to selected acupoints.

Xiao Chuan Gao (Wheezing & Dyspnea Paste) consisted of: processed Semen Sinapis Albae (_Zhi Bai Jie Zi_) and Rhizoma Corydalis Yanhusuo (_Yan Hu_), 30g @, Radix Euphorbiae Kansui (_Gan Sui_) and Herba Cum Radice Asari Sieboldi (_Xi Xin_), 15g @, Secretio Moschi Moschiferi (_She Xiang_), 1.5g, and Fructus Gleditschiae Chinensis (_Zao Jiao_) and Herba Ephedrae (_Ma Huang_), 6g @.

This formula is for the treatment of cold pattern wheezing and dyspnea. The herbs were ground into powder and divided into 3 portions. One portion was used for 1 treatment per person. One third of the powder was mixed with fresh ginger juice into a paste. This was made into flat cakes 5cm in diameter and applied to _Bai Lao_ (M-HN-30), _Fei Shu_ (Bl 13), and _Gao Huang_ (Bl 43) bilaterally. These were held in place with an adhesive plaster and left in place for 4-6 hours. The areas upon which these plasters have been placed should feel a burning warmth or aching and itching. When the plaster is removed, there should be erythema, warmth, or itching. This paste was applied once every 10 days or 3 times per month. The treatment was continued repeatedly for 3 years.

Fu Fang Ma Dou Ling Gao (Compound Formula Aristolochia Paste) consisted of: Fructus Aristolochiae (_Ma Dou Ling_), 9g, Radix Glycyrrhizae (_Sheng Gan Cao_), 6g, Semen Gingkonis Bilobae (_Bai Guo_), 30g, Semen Oryzae Sativae (_Jing Mi_), 45g, Folium Ilicis Cornutae (_Ju Gu Ye_), 90g, and Semen Lepidii (_Ting Li Zi_), 30g.

This plaster is for the treatment of hot pattern wheezing and dyspnea. These medicinals were ground into a fine powder and mixed into a paste with 100ml of saline solution. The resulting paste was divided into 6 even amounts and formed into flat cakes. These were applied to _Bai Lao_ (M-HN-30), _Fei Shu_ (Bl 13), and _Ge Shu_ (Bl 17) bilaterally and held in place with an adhesive plaster. The patients were treated 1 time every 10 days, 3 times per month and the application was continued for 3 years.

Zhi Chuan Gao (Stop Wheezing Paste) consisted of: Semen Sinapis Albae (*Bai Jie Zi*), Rhizoma Pinelliae Ternatae (*Fa Ban Xia*), and Cortex Cinnamomi (*Gui Xin*), 15g @, Rhizoma Corydalis Yanhusuo (*Yan Hu*), 12g, and Lignum Aquilariae Agallochae (*Chen Xiang*) and Radix Euphorbiae Kansui (*Gan Sui*), 3g @.

This plaster was used if the other two plasters had been tried with no success or if hot and cold were not obviously distinguishable. The medicinals were ground into powder and pounded into a mash with aged Rhizoma Zingiberis Officinalis (*Jiang*). This was applied to *Fei Shu* (Bl 13), *Feng Men* (Bl 12), and *Jue Yin Shu* (Bl 14) bilaterally. This paste was held in place with *Ji Dan Gao* (Chicken Egg Plaster). This dressing was applied for 12 hours and then removed. New plasters were applied each 12 hours for a total of 3 times.

Of the 610 cases of cold wheezing, 110 (23%) experienced complete cure; 380 (56%), marked improvement; 95 (15%), some improvement; and 25 (6%), no improvement. Of the 150 cases of hot wheezing, 50 (33%) experienced complete cure; 30 (20%), marked improvement; 60 (40%), some improvement; and 10 (7%), no improvement. And of the 40 cases categorized as other, 20 (50%) experienced complete cure; 10 (25%), marked improvement; 5 (12.5%), some improvement; and 5 (12.5%), no improvement. Further, of the 275 cases of light wheezing, 96% registered improvement. Of the 400 moderate cases of wheezing, 93% registered improvement. And of the 125 cases of serious wheezing, 87% registered improvement.

Cough

"When Should Herba Ephedrae (*Ma Huang*) Be Used to Arrest Cough?" by Chen Ruan-chun, *Zhong Yi Za Zhi (The Journal of Traditional Chinese Medicine)*, #5, 1993, p. 312; CC

Herba Ephedrae (*Ma Huang*) is an important medicinal for arresting cough and levelling asthma. In clinical usage it is combined with other assisting medicinals and is indicated for old and young alike. In general, it can be said that for wind cold cough and expectoration *San Ao Tang Jia Wei* (Three Unbinding Decoction with Added Flavors) may be used: Herba Ephedrae (*Ma Huang*), Semen Pruni Armeniacae (*Xing Ren*), Radix Glycyrrhizae (*Gan Cao*), Radix Peucedani (*Qian Hu*), Radix Platycodi Grandiflori (*Jie Geng*), and Folium Perillae Frutescentis (*Su Ye*). While for wind heat cough, *Ma Xing Gan Shi Tang Jia Wei* (Ephedra, Armeniaca, Licorice & Gypsum Decoction with Added Flavors) may be used: Herba Ephedrae (*Ma Huang*), Semen Pruni Armeniacae (*Xing Ren*), Radix Glycyrrhizae (*Gan Cao*), Gypsum (*Shi Gao*), Cortex Radicis Mori (*Sang Pi*), and Radix Scutellariae Baicalensis (*Huang Qin*). And if wind cold lodges in the lungs with copious clear and runny phlegm, *Xiao Qing Long Tang* (Minor Blue-green Dragon Decoction) is typically used.

Nevertheless, it is important to pay attention to the following issues. First is the question of the appropriate dose of Ephedra. Ephedra is a pungent, warm, and dissipating medicinal that diffuses and opens the flesh at the exterior. In general, a mild dose of 3-6g is indicated, and the use of more than that in the elderly or the very young is not appropriate. If the dosage of this medicinal is excessively large, not only will this not arrest the cough, but it will, more often than not, damage the lung qi. In trying to be clever, one will only out-smart oneself.

Secondly, Ephedra treats wind cold cough and expectoration and should be combined with Radix Peucedani (*Qian Hu*), Radix Platycodi Grandiflori (*Jie Geng*), or Folium Perillae Frutescentis (*Su Ye*) to assist the Ephedra in diffusing the lung qi. In this case, it is inappropriate to use cool or cold medicinals such as Herba Houttuyniae Cordatae (*Yu Xing Cao*). Some people combine 10g of Ephedra with 30g of Houttuynia and call this "anti-inflammatory". These formulations are most often ineffective and such combinations are inappropriate. It is a mistake to perceive all coughs as bronchitis and assume that heat must be cleared from all inflammations. The strength of Ephedra's being pungent and warm, diffusing the lungs and arresting cough is attenuated by cool and cold (medicinals), and they make it difficult for the functions of diffusion and dissipation to be given free reign. If a small amount of Ephedra is used and combined with other medicinals for diffusing the lungs, the result will be better.

Third, a clinical indicator for the use of Ephedra in arresting cough is the presence of the symptom of scratchy throat. If this scratchy throat produces cough and is more pronounced in the afternoon and evening, this is wind cold lodging in the lungs and inhibiting the lung qi. (This condition) does not rule out Ephedra's pungent, warm, diffusing and dispersing capacity. In this case, one may combine Ephedra with an appropriate dose of medicinals for diffusing the lungs for a positive therapeutic effect.

"The Treatment of 38 Cases of Cough with *Xiao Chai Hu Tang Jia Jian* (Minor Bupleurum Decoction with Additions & Subtractions)" by Liu Ming-hao, *Shang Hai Zhong Yi Yao Za Zhi (The Shanghai Journal of Traditional Chinese Medicine & Medicinals)*, #1, 1994, p. 19; BF

In this clinical report, 38 patients with cough were treated with *Xiao Chai Hu Tang Jia Jian*. Of these 38, 22 were men and 16 were women. Eight cases were between 16-30 years of age, 10 cases between 31-40, 14 cases between 41-60, and 6 cases were more than 60 years old. Twenty-seven patients had been ill from between 8-14 days, 6 between 15-21 days, and 5 for 22 days or more. Twenty-nine cases had a temperature 38° C or below, 7 cases between 38.1-39° C, and 2 cases 39° C or above. All had taken modern Western medicinals but without effect and their upper respiratory tract infections remained uncured. They were diagnosed according to TCM as displaying a righteous vacuity, evil repletion pattern. Their symptoms included cough with copious phlegm which was either white colored and pasty or clear and watery, fever, chest and lateral costal aching and pain, occasional itch in the throat, and a weak body and lack of strength. Their tongues were pale or pale red and their edges had tooth indentations. Their pulse was floating and fine or fine and wiry.

The formula used consisted of: Radix Bupleuri (*Chai Hu*), 9g, Rhizoma Pinelliae Ternatae (*Ban Xia*), 9g, Radix Scutellariae Baicalensis (*Huang Qin*), 9g, Radix Codonposis Pilosulae (*Dang Shen*), 12-30g (or Herba Agrimoniae Pilosae [*Xian He Cao*], the same amount), Radix Glycyrrhizae (*Gan Cao*), 4.5g, raw Rhizoma Zingiberis (*Sheng Jiang*), 3 slices, Cortex Magnoliae Officinalis (*Chuan Pu*), 9g, Semen Pruni Armeniacae (*Xing Ren*), 9g, and Fructus Zizyphi Jujubae (*Hong Zao*), 5 pieces.

If external invasion symptoms were heavy and the defensive yang was not aroused, Ramulus Cinnamomi (*Gui Zhi*) and Radix Albus Paeoniae Lactiflorae (*Bai Shao*), 9g @, were added. If there was cough with frothy, foamy phlegm, dry Rhizoma Zingiberis (*Gan Jiang*), 3g, Herba Cum Radice Asari Sieboldi (*Xi Xin*), 1.5g, and Fructus Schizandrae Chinensis (*Wu Wei Zi*), 9g, were added. If there was depressive heat in the lungs, Fructus Forsythiae Suspensae (*Lian Qiao*), 12g, and Rhizoma Phragmitis Communis (*Lu Gen*), 30g, were added. If there was a dry throat with worse cough in the afternoon and a desire for water which soothed (the throat and cough) accompanied by pasty, scant phlegm, fresh Ginger and Codonopsis were removed and replaced by Radix Glehniae Littoralis (*Bei Sha Shen*) and Radix Adenophorae (*Nan Sha Shen*), 12g @, plus Tuber Ophiopogonis Japonicae (*Mai Dong*), 9g.

Cure consisted of recession of the fever and stoppage of the cough within 6 days with no other obvious symptoms and a normal chest x-ray. Based on this definition, 14 cases were cured. Marked improvement consisted of recession of the fever and stoppage of the cough in 7-10 days with improvement of the chest x-ray. Based on this definition, 15 cases were markedly improved. Some improvement meant that the fever had receded and the cough was obviously diminished in 7-10 days but the chest x-ray was still not completely right. Based on these criteria, 5 patients got some improvement. Four cases experienced no result.

Trigeminal Neuralgia

"The Treatment of 28 Cases of Trigeminal Neuralgia with *San Chong Jiao Nang* (Three Insects Gelatin Capsules)" by Sun Xing-zhen & Zhang Yong-hua, *Zhe Jiang Zhong Yi Za Zhi (Zhejiang Journal of Traditional Chinese Medicine)*, #8, 1993, p. 347; BF

This is a report on the treatment of 28 cases of trigeminal neuralgia. The treatment method consisted of powdering dried Lumbricus (*Di Long*), Eupolyphaga Seu Opisthoplatia (*Di Bie Chong*), and Bombyx Batryticatus (*Jiang Can*). The resulting powder was put into empty gelatin capsules which held 0.5g @. Four such capsules were given 3 times per day. During this treatment, the administration of all other Chinese and Western medicinals were stopped as was any acupuncture/moxibustion treatment. Among the 28 patients, 15 were men and 13 were women. They ranged in age from 30-72 years of age. Their disease course had lasted from 6 months to 16 years.

After using the above medicinals from 15-30 days, 16 cases were cured, meaning that their pain had disappeared and did not return within half a year. Nine cases experienced improvement, meaning that their aching and pain had obviously diminished and the number of recurrences within the next half year were markedly less. Only 3 cases experienced no results with their condition remaining unchanged from before to after treatment. Among the cured cases, 14 were followed up 2 year later. Nine of these had experienced no relapse. Six had experienced short relapses which were immediately cured after taking _San Chong Jiao Nang_ again.

Vascular Headache

"The Treatment of 36 Cases of Vascular Headache with _Xiong Gui Si Chong San_ (Ligusticum & Dang Gui Four Insects Powder)" by Sun Jing-lan, _Zhe Jiang Zhong Yi Za Zhi (The Zhejiang Journal of Traditional Chinese Medicine)_, #10, 1993, p. 449; BF

Since 1986, the author has treated 36 cases of vascular headache with _Xiong Gui Si Chong San_. Of these 36, 11 were men and 25 were women. They ranged in age from a high of 64 to a low of 17 years old. The longest course of disease was 16 years and the shortest was 10 months. Seven cases suffered from frontal headache, 3 from one-sided headache, 6 from pain at the vertex, 3 from occipital pain, 2 from movable pain, and the rest from bilateral headaches. Other conditions members of this study also complained of were insomnia, tinnitus, toothache, a bitter taste in their mouths, and constipation.

Xiong Gui So Chong San consists of: Rhizoma Ligustici Wallichii (_Chuan Xiong_), Radix Angelicae Sinensis (_Dang Gui_), and Radix Angelicae (_Bai Zhi_), 12g @, Herba Cum Radix Asari Sieboldi (_Xi Xin_), 3g, Buthus Martensis (_Quan Xie_) and Bombyx Batryticatus

(*Jiang Can*), 10g @, Lumbricus (*Di Long*), 6-10g, Scolopendra Subspinipes (*Wu Gong*), 2-3 pieces, and Fructus Piperis Longi (*Bi Ba*), 10g. If there was insomnia, Semen Zizyphi Spinosae (*Suan Zao Ren*), 30g, was added. If there was ringing in the ears and a bitter mouth, Radix Gentianae Scabrae (*Long Dan Cao*), 10g, was added. If there was toothache, Gypsum (*Shi Gao*), 30g, was added. If there was constipation, raw Radix Et Rhizoma Rhei (*Sheng Da Huang*), 10g, was added. If the tongue coating was comparatively thick and phlegm dampness was obvious, Rhizoma Pinelliae Ternatae (*Ban Xia*), 12g, and bile(-processed) Rhizoma Arisaematis (*Dan Xing*), 6-10g, were added. These medicinals were decocted in 300ml of water and taken in two equal doses, 1 *ji* per day. If the cases were serious, 2 *ji* per day were administered. Nine days equalled 1 course of treatment. If these medicinals were taken and there was some resolution of the symptoms, the formula was administered for another course of treatment. However, if after 1 course of treatment there was no change in the symptoms, treatment was discontinued and this was defined as no result.

Fifteen cases, or 42%, were completely cured using this protocol. This meant that their symptoms disappeared and there was no recurrence on follow-up after 1 year. Eighteen cases or 50% received some improvement. This meant that their headaches stopped after taking these medicinals but when these medicinals were discontinued their headaches returned. Three cases or 8% got no result from this treatment. Therefore, the combined amelioration rate was 92%.

According to the author, vascular headaches are due to bandit wind taking advantage of blood vacuity. This then results in qi stagnation and blood stasis. Therefore, the treatment principles are to dispel wind and track down (wind in) the connecting vessels, quicken the blood and open the connecting vessels. Within this formula, Ligusticum, Angelica, and Asarum dispel wind and stop pain. Ligusticum and *Dang Gui* nourish and quicken the blood. Scorpion, Silkworm, Earthworm, and Centipede track down wind and open the connecting vessels, resolve convulsions and stop pain. According to the _Ben Cao Gang Mu (The Complete Outline of Materia Medica)_, Piper Longus is an essential herb for the treatment of headache. Thus these medicinals in combination dispel wind and open the connecting vessels, quicken the blood and stop pain. However, in clinical practice, if this condition relapses due to pathological emotional activity, it may require the use of double the amounts of medicine.

Obesity

"The Treatment of Obesity Based on Pattern Discrimination" by Zhao Huai-cong, _Si Chuan Zhong Yi (Sichuan Traditional Chinese Medicine)_, #8, 1993, p. 9-10; BF

The author of this short essay does not give any statistics or case histories as evidence in support of their thesis. Nonetheless, this material may prove useful to some clinicians.

1. Spleen loss of healthy movement, phlegm dampness accumulating internally

The signs and symptoms of this pattern include reduced appetite, a fatigued spirit and lack of strength, chest and upper abdominal oppression, excessive phlegm, a white, slimy tongue coating, and a sodden, slippery pulse. In this case, the treatment principles are to transform phlegm and disinhibit dampness. The formula to use is _Ping Wei San_ (Level the Stomach Powder) combined with _Er Chen Tang Jia Jian_ (Two Aged [Ingredients] Decoction with Additions & Subtractions): Pericarpium Citri Reticulatae (_Chen Pi_), Rhizoma Atractylodis (_Cang Zhu_), Cortex Magnoliae Officinalis (_Hou Po_), Rhizoma Pinelliae Ternatae (_Ban Xia_), Yunnan Sclerotium Poriae Cocos (_Yun Ling_), Rhizoma Atractylodis Macrocephalae (_Bai Zhu_), Rhizoma Alismatis (_Ze Xie_), etc.

2. Yang qi insufficiency

The clinical manifestations of this pattern include low back pain, soreness, and heaviness, short, scanty urination, fear of cold and fatigued spirit, an ashen, stagnant facial color, a pale, fat tongue with a white coating, and a deep, fine pulse. The treatment principles are to warm yang and disinhibit water. The formula to use is *Ji Sheng Shen Qi Wan* (Abundant Life Kidney Qi Pills) combined with *Ling Gui Zhu Gan Tang Jia Jian* (Poria, Cinnamon, Atractylodes, & Licorice Decoction with Additions & Subtractions): prepared Radix Rehmanniae (*Shu Di*), Radix Dioscoreae Oppositae (*Shan Yao*), Fructus Corni Officinalis (*Zhu Rou*), Yunnan Sclerotium Poriae Cocos (*Yun Ling*), Radix Praeparatus Aconiti Carmichaeli (*Fu Zi*), Rhizoma Alismatis (*Ze Xie*), Ramulus Cinnamomi (*Gui Zhi*), Radix Achyranthis Bidentatae (*Niu Xi*), Semen Plantaginis (*Che Qian Zi*), Rhizoma Atractylodis Macrocephalae (*Bai Zhu*), etc.

3. Liver depression, qi stagnation

The clinical manifestations of this pattern include lateral costal and rib distention and pain, chest oppression aggravated by emotional stress, belching, and a wiry pulse. The treatment principles are to course the liver and disinhibit the gallbladder. The formula to use is *Chai Hu Shu Gan Tang* (Bupleurum Course the Liver Decoction) combined with *Jin Ling Zi San Jia Jian* (Melia Powder with Additions & Subtractions): Radix Bupleuri (*Chai Hu*), Rhizoma Cyperi Rotundi (*Xiang Fu*), Fructus Citri Seu Ponciri (*Zhi Ke*), Tuber Curcumae (*Yu Jin*), Fructus Meliae Toosendan (*Chuan Lian Zi*), Rhizoma Corydalis Yanhusuo (*Yan Hu*), Herba Menthae (*Bo He*), etc.

4. Food & drink loss of discipline, stopping and gathering in the center

The symptoms of this pattern include abdominal distention and oppression, belching and sour eructation, constipation, and a thick, slimy tongue coating. The treatment principles are to disperse food and conduct stagnation. The formula to use is *Xiao Cheng Qi Tang* (Minor Order the Qi Decoction) combined with *Bao He Wan Jia Jian* (Protect Harmony Pills with Additions & Subtractions): Radix Et Rhizoma Rhei (*Da Huang*), Cortex Magnoliae Officinalis (*Hou Po*), Fructus Immaturus Citri Seu Ponciri (*Zhi Shi*), Semen Arecae Catechu (*Bing Lang*), Fructus Crataegi (*Shan Zha*), Rhizoma Pinelliae Ternatae (*Ban Xia*), Massa Medica Fermentata (*Shen Qu*), Semen Raphani Sativi (*Lai Fu Zi*), etc.

In addition to taking the above medicinals, one must also regulate their activity and reduce the amount of food they eat and especially fats and sweets. They should also get more exercise and stabilize their emotions.

Colitis

"The Pattern Discrimination Treatment of 40 Cases of Ulcerative Colitis" by Li Xiu-yun, *Si Chuan Zhong Yi (Sichuan Traditional Chinese Medicine)*, #11, 1993, p. 32; BF

Beginning from 1984, the author has treated 40 cases of this disease based on pattern discrimination assisted by Chinese herbal retention enemas. Of these 40 cases, 28 were men and 12 were women. Four were between 21-30 years of age, 24 between 31-40, 10 between 41-50, and 2 were 51 years old or more. The longest course of disease was 10 years and the shortest was 1 month, with most patients having suffered with this condition for 3-5 years. Pattern discrimination was based on signs and symptoms, and tongue and pulse images.

1. Stomach & intestine damp heat pattern (15 cases)

Qing Wei Bai Du San (Clear the Stomach & Defeat Toxins Powder; the translator has not been able to identify the ingredients of this formula) was used to clear and discharge the *yang ming*, regulate the qi and harmonize the stomach. If heat toxins were severe, Radix Pulsatillae (*Bai Tou Weng*), Cortex Phellodendri (*Huang Bai*), Cortex Fraxini (*Qin Pi*), and Cortex Radicis Moutan (*Dan Pi*) were added. If damp turbidity was heavy, Rhizoma Atractylodis (*Cang Zhu*), Herba Agastachis Seu Pogostemi (*Huo Xiang*), etc. were added. If abdominal pain was severe, Rhizoma Corydalis Yanhusuo (*Yuan Hu*) and Radix Albus Paeoniae Lactiflorae (*Bai Shao*) were added. Afterwards, *Liu Jun Zi Tang* (Six Gentlemen Decoction) was given to aid recuperation.

2. Liver depression, qi stagnation, spleen vacuity pattern (12 cases)

In order to course the liver and rectify the qi, strengthen the spleen and boost the qi, *Tong Xie Yao Fang* (Essential Formula for Painful Diarrhea) was given. If there was liver depression with effulgent fire, Fructus Gardeniae Jasminoidis (*Shan Zhi*), Cortex Radicis Moutan (*Dan Pi*), Radix Bupleuri (*Chai Hu*), Radix Angelicae Sinensis (*Dang Gui*), etc. were added in order to course the liver and resolve depression, drain the liver and supplement the spleen. If there were loose stools, Sclerotium Poriae Cocos (*Fu Ling*) and Rhizoma Atractylodis Macrocephalae (*Bai Zhu*) were added. *Gui Shao Liu Jun Zi Tang* (Peony & *Dang Gui* Six Gentlemen Decoction was given to aid recuperation.

3. Spleen & stomach qi vacuity pattern (10 cases)

Patients were administered *Pi Wei Shuang Bu Wan* (Spleen & Stomach Dual Supplementing Pills): Radix Astragali Membranacei (*Huang Qi*), Radix Codonopsis Pilosulae (*Dang Shen*), and mix-fried Radix Glycyrrhizae (*Zhi Gan Cao*), 15g @, Rhizoma Atractylodis Macroce-phalae (*Bai Zhu*), Rhizoma Corydalis Yanhusuo (*Yuan Hu*), Hallyosi-tum Rubrum (*Chi Shi Zhi*), Acacia Catechu (*Er Cha*), and Radix Albus Paeoniae Lactiflorae (*Bai Shao*), 10g @, Cortex Cinnamomi (*Rou Gui*, stirred in at the end of decocting the other medicinals) and

Semen Litchi Sinensis (*Li Zhi He*), 4g @, Fructus Amomi (*Sha Ren*), Radix Angelicae Sinensis (*Dang Gui*), Radix Saussureae Seu Vladimiriae (*Guang Mu Xiang*), blast-fried Rhizoma Zingiberis (*Pao Jiang*), and Radix Ledebouriellae Sesloidis (*Fang Feng*), and Sclerotium Poriae Cocos (*Fu Ling*), 12g.

4. Spleen, stomach & kidney yang vacuity pattern (3 cases)

Patients were administered *Si Shen Wan* (Four Spirits Pills) combined with *Fu Zi Li Zhong Wan* (Aconite Rectify the Center Pills) in the form of a decoction in order to supplement the source yang. In old patients with deficient bodies (*i.e.*, constitutions), for qi vacuity with downward falling, or for long-term ceaseless diarrhea, Radix Codonopsis Pilosulae (*Dang Shen*), Radix Astragali Membranacei (*Huang Qi*), Rhizoma Atractylodis Macrocephalae (*Bai Zhu*), Rhizoma Cimicifugae (*Sheng Ma*), Radix Praeparatus Aconiti Carmichaeli (*Fu Zi*), Cortex Cinnamomi (*Rou Gui*), and blast-fried Rhizoma Zingiberis (*Pao Jiang*) were added to boost the qi, warm yang, and secure and astringe.

In all the above patterns, in order to resolve the bloody stools, the following retention enema was administered 1 time per day: Radix Sophorae Flavescentis (*Ku Shen*), 30g, Radix Sanguisorbae (*Di Yu*), 15g, Radix Polygoni Bistortae (*Zi Shen*) and Galla Rhi Chinensis (*Wu Pei Zi*), 10g @, Rhizoma Coptidis Chinensis (*Huang Lian*), 6g, and Cortex Phellodendri (*Huang Bai*), 12g. These were decocted in 100ml of water.

After 2-3 months of treatment, 4 cases were completely cured, 29 were obviously improved, 6 experienced some improvement, and 1 experienced no results for a combined amelioration rate of 95%.

"A Clinical Report on the Treatment of 42 Cases of Chronic Colitis" by Ni Ke-zhong & Peng Mei-yu, *Shang Hai Zhong Yi Yao Za Zhi (Shanghai Journal of Chinese Medicine)*, #11, 1993, p. 19-20; BF

From 1989-1992, the authors saw 56 cases of chronic colitis. Of these, 42 cases were treated for a full 3 months. Among this latter group, 19 were men and 23 were women. Seven cases ranged in age between 20-30 years, 18 between 31-40, 13 between 41-50, and 4 cases were 51 years old or older. Eighteen cases had suffered for from 1-5 years and 24 cases from 6-10 years. In addition, 30 cases had bowel movements 3-5 times per day and 12 cases 6-10 times per day. Seventeen cases had pasty, gelatinous stools and 8 had bright-colored blood. Forty-two cases had borborygmus and abdominal pain, and 27 had post-defecatory tenesmus. Eight cases had a thin, white tongue coating, 29 cases a thin, yellow, slimy coating, and 5 cases a yellow, slimy coating. Twelve patients' tongues were pale, 17 slightly red, and 13 light red. Twenty-four had fine, rapid pulses, 8 had fine, wiry pulses, and 10 had fine pulses. In all, 11 patients were diagnosed by TCM as liver/spleen not harmonious pattern and 31 cases as spleen vacuity and damp heat pattern.

1. Liver/spleen not harmonious pattern

The signs and symptoms of this pattern consisted of borborygmus, abdominal pain, and diarrhea with pain relieved after diarrhea, a thin, white tongue coating and pale tongue, and a fine, wiry pulse. Internal medication for this pattern consisted of: Radix Bupleuri (*Chai Hu*), 6g, Radix Albus Paeoniae Lactiflorae (*Bai Shao*), 30g, Pericarpium Citri Reticulatae (*Chen Pi*), 6g, Fructus Citri Seu Ponciri (*Zhi Ke*), 6g, Rhizoma Atractylodis Macrocephalae (*Bai Zhu*), 10g, Fructus Meliae Toosendanis (*Chuan Lian Zi*), 10g, Rhizoma Corydalis Yanhusuo (*Yan Hu Suo*), 10g, Herba Portulacae Oleraceae (*Ma Chi Xian*), 30g, and Fructus Chaenomelis Lagenariae (*Mu Gua*), 10g; 1 *ji* per day.

2. Spleen vacuity, damp heat pattern

The signs and symptoms of this pattern consisted of borborygmus, abdominal pain, pasty, gelatinous stools, torpid intake, exhausted spirit, lack of strength, a sallow, yellowish facial complexion, and a bitter, dry mouth, a thin, yellow, slimy or yellow, slimy tongue coating, either a slightly red or light red tongue, and a soggy, fine, rapid pulse. Internal medication for this pattern consisted of: Radix Puerariae (_Ge Gen_), 10g, Radix Dioscoreae Oppositae (_Shan Yao_), 30g, Radix Paeoniae Lactiflorae (_Shao Yao_), 30g, Rhizoma Coptidis Chinensis (_Huang Lian_), 6g, blast-fried Rhizoma Zingiberis (_Pao Jiang_), 10g, Radix Scutellariae Baicalensis (_Huang Qin_), 10g, Herba Portulacae Oleraceae (_Ma Chi Xian_), 30g, raw Radix Sanguisorbae (_Sheng Di Yu_), 12g, stir-fried Flos Lonicerae Japonicae (_Chao Yin Hua_), 10g, and Semen Plantaginis (_Che Qian Zi_, wrapped), 10g; 1 _ji_ per day.

External treatment consisted of a Chinese herbal retention enema whose ingredients were: Herba Portulacae Oleraceae (_Ma Chi Xian_), 30g, Caulis Sargentodoxae (_Hong Teng_), 30g, and Rhizoma Coptidis Chinensis (_Huang Lian_), 6g. These were decocted in 100cc of water. Two grams of _Xi Lei San_ were stirred in after the other ingredients were decocted. (_Xi Lei San_ is a patent medicine. Literally, its name translates as tin-like powder. Its ingredients consist of: Bezoar [_Niu Huang_], Borneol [_Bing Pian_], Margarita [_Zhen Zhu_], human nails [_Ren Zhi Jia_], Dens Elephantis [_Xiang Ya Si_], Pulvis Indigonis [_Qing Dai_], and Uroctea Compactilis [_Bi Qian_, a spider]. This patent medicine was originally developed to treat putrefaction of the throat and swelling and pain of the lips and tongue.)

Four weeks' use of the above medicinals equalled 1 course of treatment. After each course, treatment was suspended for 5-7 days before commencing a new course. Clinical results were based on 3 whole courses of treatment. Complete cure was defined as disappearance of the condition's symptoms, normal stools, and no relapse on follow-up a half year later. Improvement was defined as improvement in symptoms with bowel movements reduced to 2-3 times per day. No improvement was defined as either no change in symptoms or a worsening of the condition. Based on these criteria, 17 were cured, 21 experienced improvement, and 4 no improvement.

According to the authors, chronic colitis is called diarrhea (*xie xie*), intestinal wind (*chang feng*), downward dysentery (*xia li*), etc. in TCM. The causes of this disease are divided between wind, cold, dampness, heat, and stasis. However, according to Zhang Jing-yue in his *Jing Yue Quan Shu (Complete Writings of Jing-yue)*, "The root of diarrhea is nothing other than the spleen and stomach." Eating unclean food may lead to food stagnation and transformative heat. Damp heat evils may then accumulate in the large intestine. In that case, the large intestine's conduction and conveyance do not do their duty and clearing and discharging are not separated. This may give rise to acute diarrhea, which, if it is not treated in a timely manner, may become chronic. In this case, prolonged injury and damage to the spleen and stomach's transportation and transformation may result in their not doing their duty. This may then give rise to chronic diarrhea which, over time, becomes difficult to cure. It is also possible for invasion of cold or overtaxation to cause spleen and stomach vacuity weakness. If their transportation and transformation do not do their duty, dampness and heat may accumulate in the large intestine. Thus, in this condition, there is usually vacuity but mixed with repletion. Although this disease is situated in the large intestine in the lower burner, the root of this disease comes from the two viscera, the liver and spleen, in the middle burner. Therefore, one must treat both these burners at the same time.

The authors feel that, in the treatment of this disease, the combined use of internally administered and externally applied Chinese herbal medicinals (*i.e.*, retention enemas) achieve a better result than using internally administered decoctions orally alone. Once the bowel movements become normal, both the internal and external medicinals should not be stopped too soon since this condition may easily relapse. Thus one should not stop treatment before 1 whole course has been administered. Further, after the bowel movements have become normal, one should continue boosting the qi and strengthening the spleen since the spleen is the latter heaven root of the origin of generation and transformation. Therefore, one can use either _Shen Ling Bai Zhu San_ (Ginseng, Poria & Atractylodes Powder) or _Liu Jun Zi Tang_ (Six Gentlemen Decoction) with additions and subtractions.

"The Treatment of 25 Cases of Chronic Ulcerative Colitis by the Methods of Boosting the Qi and Quickening the Blood" by Chen De-jiao, _Zhe Jiang Zhong Yi Za Zhi (Zhejiang Journal of Traditional Chinese Medicine)_, #10, 1993, p. 443; BF

Chronic ulcerative colitis is one of the most commonly seen conditions in internal medicine departments. It is characterized by abdominal pain and diarrhea with a mucoid discharge or bloody stools. It frequently recurs and is difficult to cure. The author of this study reports on their treatment of 25 cases of chronic ulcerative colitis using the methods of boosting the qi and quickening the blood combined with TCM pattern discrimination. Of the 25 cases, 16 were men and 9 were women. Their ages ranged from 23-58 years old, with 2 cases between 23-30, 6 cases between 31-40, 13 cases between 41-50, and 4 cases 51 years of age or older. The longest course of disease was 6 years and most cases had suffered with this condition for over 1 year. Everyone in this study had been diagnosed with ulcerative colitis by modern Western medicine. Typically, the disease recurred and receded based on whether these patients were relaxed or tense emotionally.

1. Spleen vacuity, damp heat pattern

Treatment consisted of boosting the qi and strengthening the spleen, quickening the blood, clearing heat, and stopping diarrhea. The formula used was *Bu Zhong Yi Qi Tang* (Supplement the Center & Boost the Qi Decoction) combined with *Bai Tou Weng Tang Jia Jian* (Pulsatilla Decoction with Additions & Subtractions). The medicinals used were: Radix Codonopsis Pilosulae (*Dang Shen*), Radix Astragali Membranacei (*Huang Qi*), Sclerotium Poriae Cocos (*Fu Ling*), Rhizoma Atractylodis Macrocephalae (*Bai Zhu*), Cortex Magnoliae Officinalis (*Hou Po*), Radix Saussureae Seu Vladimiriae (*Guang Mu Xiang*), Cortex Radicis Moutan (*Dan Pi*), Radix Rubrus Paeoniae Lactiflorae (*Chi Shao*), Radix Pulsatillae (*Bai Tou Weng*), Rhizoma Corydalis Yanhusuo (*Xuan Hu*), and Radix Angelicae Sinensis (*Dang Gui*). If abdominal pain was severe, Radix Albus Paeoniae Lactiflorae (*Bai Shao*) was added. If there was bloody stools, carbonized Radix Sanguisorbae (*Di Yu Tan*) and carbonized Radix Et Rhizoma Rhei (*Da Huang Tan*) were added.

2. Spleen/kidney yang vacuity pattern

This was treated by warming the kidneys and strengthening the spleen, quickening the blood and moving the qi. The formula used was *Bu Zhong Yi Qi Tang* combined with *Si Shen Wan Jia Jian* (Four Spirits Pills with Additions & Subtractions). The medicinals used were: Radix Codonopsis Pilosulae (*Dang Shen*), Radix Astragali Membranacei (*Huang Qi*), Sclerotium Poriae Cocos (*Fu Ling*), Rhizoma Atractylodis Macrocephalae (*Bai Zhu*), Radix Angelicae Sinensis (*Dang Gui*), Fructus Psoraleae Corylifoliae (*Bu Gu Zhi*), Semen Myristicae Fragrantis (*Rou Dou Kou*), Radix Praeparatus Aconiti Carmichaeli (*Fu Pian*), and blast-fried Rhizoma Zingiberis (*Pao Jiang*). If diarrhea was prolonged with qi vacuity and downward prolapse, large amounts of Codonopsis and Astragalus were used. If there was tenesmus and pain, Fructus Foeniculi Vulgaris (*Xiao Hui*) was added. If grains were not being transformed, parched Fructus Crataegi (*Jiao Zha*) was added. If there was a white colored, mucoid discharge with the stools, Rhizoma Atractylodis (*Cang Zhu*) was added.

3. Qi & yin dual vacuity pattern

The treatment for this pattern consisted of boosting the qi and nourishing yin, cooling the blood, quickening the blood, and stopping diarrhea. The medicinals used were: Radix Codonopsis Pilosulae (*Dang Shen*), Radix Astragali Membranacei (*Huang Qi*), Sclerotium Poriae Cocos (*Fu Ling*), raw Radix Rehmanniae (*Sheng Di*), Cortex Radicis Moutan (*Dan Pi*), Radix Rubrus Paeoniae Lactiflorae (*Chi Shao*), Fructus Schizandrae Chinensis (*Wu Wei Zi*), Tuber Ophiopogonis Japonicae (*Mai Dong*), and Cortex Phellodendri (*Huang Bai*). If there was abdominal pain, Radix Albus Paeoniae Lactiflorae (*Bai Shao*) and Rhizoma Corydalis Yanhusuo (*Xuan Hu*) were added. And if there was a mucoid discharge and bloody stools, carbonized Radix Et Rhizoma Rhei (*Da Huang Tan*) was added.

Of the 25 patients treated with this protocol, 5 cases experienced marked improvement. This meant that their symptoms disappeared, their stools returned to normal, and that their colonoscopy was normal. Eighteen cases got good improvement. This meant that their clinical symptoms were obviously diminished and that the number of bowel movements was reduced. And 2 cases experienced no result, their symptoms and colonoscopy remaining unchanged.

The author states that this disease may remain unhealed even after prolonged treatment. This is because prolonged disease enters the connecting vessels, causing stasis and stagnation of the qi and blood. Thus there is diarrhea with abdominal pain and bloody stools with mucoid discharge. Although the site of this disease is in the intestines, it is due to spleen vacuity internally engendering dampness. If this remains, it may cause chronic depression and gathering transforming into heat. This then becomes damp heat in the intestinal tract which damages the connecting vessels and causes ulceration. Therefore, in this condition, it is necessary to support the righteous and strengthen the spleen but also to quicken the blood and transform stasis while simultaneously using astringing and restraining substances.

Plum Pit Qi

"An Explanation of the Pattern Discrimination Treatment of 49 Cases of Plum Pit Qi" by Yuan Chang-hua, *Si Chuan Zhong Yi (Sichuan Traditional Chinese Medicine)*, #11, 1993, p. 33-4; BF

This clinical audit describes the treatment of 49 cases of plum pit qi (*mei he qi*). Of these 49 cases, 13 were men and 36 women. Their ages ranged from a high of 76 to a low of 18 years old. The course of their disease had lasted from as long as 3 years to as short as 2 weeks. Treatment was given on the basis of a pattern discrimination diagnosis with four patterns being identified.

1. Liver depression, qi stagnation pattern

The signs and symptoms of this pattern included the sensation of something stuck in the throat which could neither be coughed up and out nor descended by swallowing, chest and lateral costal distention and pain, emotional lability, deep sighing, violent anger, a thin, white tongue coating, and wiry pulse. The treatment methods were to course the liver and resolve depression, rectify the qi and scatter nodulation. The formula used was *Si Ni San Jia Jian* (Four Counterflows Powder with Additions and Subtractions).

The formula consisted of: Radix Bupleuri (*Chai Hu*), Fructus Immaturus Citri Seu Ponciri (*Zhi Shi*), Radix Paeoniae Lactiflorae from Hangzhou (*Hang Shao*), Tuber Curcumae (*Yu Jin*), Caulis Perillae Frutescentis (*Su Geng*), Rhizoma Cyperi Rotundi (*Xiang Fu*), Radix Platycodi Grandiflori (*Jie Geng*), etc. If liver depression transformed into fire, Cortex Radicis Moutan (*Dan Pi*), Fructus Gardeniae Jasminoidis (*Zhi Zi*), Spica Prunellae Vulgaris (*Xia Gu Cao*), Fructus Meliae Toosendan (*Chuan Lian Zi*), etc. were added.

2. Phlegm depression in the chest & diaphragm pattern

The signs and symptoms of this pattern included a feeling of phlegm stuck in the throat which would neither go down with swallowing or be discharged upward by cough, distention and oppression of the chest and diaphragm, a pasty, slimy feeling in the mouth, possible nausea and vomiting, a thick, slimy tongue coating, and a wiry, slippery pulse. The treatment methods were to transform phlegm, rectify the qi, and scatter nodulation. The formula used was *Ban Xia Hou Po Tang Jia Jian* (Pinellia & Magnolia Decoction with Additions & Subtractions).

The formula consisted of: Rhizoma Pinelliae Ternatae (*Ban Xia*), Cortex Magnoliae Officinalis (*Chuan Po*), Sclerotium Poriae Cocos from Yunnan (*Yun Ling*), Radix Platycodi Grandiflori (*Jie Geng*), Caulis Perillae Frutescentis (*Su Geng*), Semen Sinapis Albae (*Bai Jie Zi*), Tuber Curcumae (*Yu Jin*), Radix Clematidis Chinensis (*Ling Xian*), Fructus Immaturus Citri Seu Ponciri (*Zhi Shi*), etc. If there was also a bitter taste in the mouth and coughing of yellow, sticky phlegm, dizziness, a slimy, yellow tongue coating, and a slippery, rapid pulse, then *Wen Dan Tang Jia Jian* (Warm the Gallbladder Decoction with Additions & Subtractions) was the formula used, consisting of: Rhizoma Pinelliae Ternatae (*Ban Xia*), Pericarpium Citri Reticulatae (*Chen Pi*), Sclerotium Poriae Cocos from Yunnan (*Yun Ling*), Fructus Immaturus Citri Seu Ponciri (*Zhi Shi*), Caulis In Taeniis Bambusae (*Zhu Ru*), Fructus Trichosanthis Kirlowii (*Gua Lou*), Bulbus Fritillariae Thunbergii (*Zhe Bei*), Tuber Curcumae (*Yu Jin*), Spica Prunellae Vulgaris (*Xia Gu Cao*), Radix Scutellariae Baicalensis (*Huang Qin*), Rhizoma Belamcandae (*She Gan*), etc.

3. Yin vacuity, liver depression pattern

The signs and symptoms of this pattern consisted of the sensation of something obstructing and stopping the throat which could neither be coughed out nor swallowed down, a dry mouth and throat, heat in the center of the hands and feet (or heat in the hands, feet, and heart depending on how you read the Chinese), lingering pain in the lateral costal region and ribs, a red tongue with scant coating, and a wiry, fine, and rapid pulse. The treatment methods used were to enrich yin and downbear fire, soften the liver and scatter nodulation. The formula used was *Yi Guan Jian* (Linking Decoction with Additions & Subtractions).

The formula consisted of: Fructus Meliae Toosendan (*Chuan Lian Zi*), Radix Glehniae Littoralis (*Sha Shen*), Tuber Ophiopogonis Japonicae (*Mai Dong*), raw Radix Rehmanniae (*Sheng Di Huang*), Fructus Lycii Sinensis (*Gou Qi*), Radix Angelicae Sinensis (*Dang Gui*), Radix Scrophulariae Ningpoensis (*Xuan Shen*), Tuber Curcumae (*Yu Jin*), Radix Platycodi Grandiflori (*Jie Geng*), Radix Paeoniae Lactiflorae from Hangzhou (*Hang Shao*), etc.

4. Blood stasis obstructing the connecting vessels pattern

The signs and symptoms of this pattern included the feeling of something blocking the throat which could neither be coughed up nor swallowed down, eating resulting in constipation, water drinking normal, lancinating chest and lateral costal region pain which, if serious, radiated to the upper back region, a long disease course, a dark tongue or a tongue with static spots or patches, and a wiry, fine, and choppy/astringent pulse. The treatment methods were to transform stasis and open the connecting vessels, move the qi and disinhibit the throat. The formula used was *Xue Fu Zhu Yu Tang Jia Jian* (Expel Stasis from the Mansion of the Blood Decoction with Additions & Subtractions).

The formula consisted of: Semen Pruni Persicae (*Tao Ren*), Flos Carthami Tinctorii (*Hong Hua*), Radix Angelicae Sinensis (*Dang Gui*), Rhizoma Ligustici Wallichii (*Chuan Xiong*), Radix Rubrus Paeoniae Lactiflorae (*Chi Shao*), Radix Bupleuri (*Chai Hu*), Fructus Immaturus Citri Seu Ponciri (*Zhi Shi*), Radix Platycodi Grandiflori (*Jie Geng*), Radix Cyathulae (*Chuan Xi*), Tuber Curcumae (*Yu Jin*), Spica Prunellae Vulgaris (*Xia Gu Cao*), Radix Salviae Miltiorrhizae (*Dan Shen*), etc.

The criteria for judging success in this study were as follows: Complete cure was defined as the disappearance of this condition clinically with no recurrence on follow-up one year later. Improvement consisted of disappearance of this condition clinically with recurrence within one year. And no result was defined as no obvious improvement in this condition clinically after 2 weeks of taking the above medicinals. Based on these criteria, 39 cases were completely cured, 7 cases were improved, and 3 cases experienced no improvement. This resulted in a combined amelioration rate of 93.8%.

Case history: A 42 year old woman complained of phlegm in her throat accompanied by feeling out of sorts for 3 months. She could neither cough this phlegm up nor swallow it down. In addition, she had chest oppression, inability to relax, dizziness, a bitter, sticky mouth, thirst but no desire to drink, insomnia and excessive dreams, a red tongue with a yellow, slimy coating, and a wiry, slippery pulse. The (disease) diagnosis was plum pit qi. This was categorized as phlegm depression of the chest and diaphragm pattern with phlegm and qi combining, obstructing, and transforming into heat. Treatment, therefore, was to transform phlegm and clear heat, disinhibit the qi and scatter nodulation.

The formula used was modified *Wen Dan Tang*, consisting of: Rhizoma Pinelliae Ternatae (*Ban Xia*) and Sclerotium Poriae Cocos from Yunnan (*Yun Ling*), 5g @, Pericarpium Citri Reticulatae (*Chen*

Pi), Fructus Immaturus Citri Seu Ponciri (*Zhi Shi*), Radix Scutellariae Baicalensis (*Huang Qin*), Caulis In Taeniis Bambusae (*Zhu Ru*), and Tuber Curcumae (*Yu Jin*), 10g @, Fructus Trichosanthis Kirlowii (*Gua Lou*) and Spica Prunellae Vulgaris (*Xia Gu Cao*), 30g @, Bulbus Fritillariae Thunbergii (*Zhe Bei*), 12 g, and Radix Platycodi Grandiflori (*Jie Geng*), 6g. These were decocted in water and taken, 1 *ji* per day.

After taking 3 *ji*, the patient came again for a diagnosis. The chest oppression had been diminished and her sleep was improved. The other symptoms were the same as before. Therefore, 15g of Rhizoma Belamcandae (*She Gan*) were added to the above medicinals in order to strengthen their ability to clear heat and disinhibit the throat, transform phlegm and scatter nodulation. After taking another 3 *ji* the patient was extremely happy. The throat condition was quite obviously reduced and her tongue coating had turned from yellow and glossy to thin and slimy. Therefore, there was no further change made in her formula. Three more *ji* and she was completely cured. On follow-up 1 year later, there had been no recurrence.

According to the author, plum pit qi is a disease which is mostly due to the liver and spleen. However, this disease is not limited solely to the liver and spleen but may involve the liver, stomach, spleen, kidneys, and other viscera and bowels. *Ban Xia Hou Po Tang* is the most commonly used formula for the treatment of plum pit qi. Nonetheless, because this disease may differ (in different patients), so must the formula. If treatment is not given on the basis of a pattern discrimination diagnosis, the results are not good.

Be that as it may, the author goes on to say that there are two especially important medicinals in the treatment of plum pit qi. These are Tuber Curcumae (*Yu Jin*) and Spica Prunellae Vulgaris (*Xia Gu Cao*). The *Ben Cao Hui Yan (Collected Sayings on the Materia Medica)* says of Tuber Curcumae:

Its nature should not be belittled. It is able to scatter depression and stagnation. It normalizes counterflow qi. Above, it reaches the high mountain peaks, while also moving the lower burner. (Affecting) the heart, lungs, liver, and kidneys, it is effective for even the tiniest qi, blood, phlegm, and fire depressions which are checked and not moving.

Spica Prunellae Vulgaris is bitter, acrid, and cold and enters the liver and gallbladder channels. In particular, it is able to move liver qi, open liver depression, and scatter nodulation. The _Chong Qing Chang Sui Bi (Chongqing Common Informal Essays)_ states: "Spica Prunellae Vulgaris is slightly acrid and sweet and thus scatters nodulations while at the same time harmonizing yang and nourishing yin." (Based on the above quotation,) one can understand that Spica Prunellae Vulgaris not only scatters nodulation but is also able to level the steelyard (of the hand-held scale) when regulating yin and yang. Although plum pit qi may be divided into the types described above, it is always accompanied by qi nodulation in the throat. Therefore, these two medicinals may be added when writing a formula and should be not lacking in the treatment of this disease.

"The Treatment of 40 Cases of Plum Pit Qi with _Shun Qi Xiao Shi Hua Tan Tang_ (Normalize the Qi, Disperse Food, & Transform Phlegm Decoction)" by Jin Ming-mo, _Ji Lin Zhong Yi Yao (Jilin Traditional Chinese Medicine & Medicinals)_, #4, 1993, p.19; BF

This clinical audit reports on the treatment of 40 cases of plum pit qi using _Shun Qi Xiao Shi Hua Tan Tang_ with additions and subtractions. Among these 40 cases, 12 were men and 28 were women. Ten cases ranged in age from 18-30 years old, 21 cases were 31-40 years old, 5 cases were 41-50 years old, and the rest were over 50. The course of disease had lasted from a long of 3 years to a short of 7 days.

Further, 23 cases were from emotional causes, 7 were from undisciplined diet, and the rest were due to upper respiratory tract infection.

The formula consisted of: Pericarpium Citri Reticulatae (*Chen Pi*), 10g, Pericarpium Viridis Citri Reticulatae (*Qing Pi*), 10g, bile(-treated) Rhizoma Arisaematis (*Dan Nan Xing*), 10g, Rhizoma Pinelliae Ternatae (*Ban Xia*), 10g, Fructus Perillae Frutescentis (*Su Zi*), Semen Raphani Sativi (*Lai Fu Zi*), 10g, Radix Bupleuri (*Chai Hu*), 10g, Rhizoma Cimicifugae (*Sheng Ma*), 10g, Radix Platycodi Grandiflori (*Jie Geng*), 10g, and Rhizoma Cyperi Rotundi (*Xiang Fu*), 10g. One *ji* was taken per day, decocted in water and divided into two doses.

If the emotions were not normal, Semen Biotae Orientalis (*Bai Zi Ren*), 10g, stir-fried Semen Zizyphi Spinosae (*Chao Zao Ren*), 20g, and Cortex Cinnamomi (*Gui Yuan Rou*), 10g, were added. If food and drink were not tidy and neat (*i.e.*, well regulated), Massa Medica Fermentata (*Shen Qu*), 40g, Endothelium Corneum Gigeria Galli (*Ji Nei Jin*), 10g, and stir-fried Fructus Germinatus Hordei Vulgaris (*Chao Mai Ya*), 10g, were added. If there was upper respiratory tract infection, Flos Lonicerae Japonicae (*Jin Yin Hua*), 20g, Radix Isatidis Seu Baphicacanthis (*Ban Lang Gen*), 50g, and Herba Cum Radice Taraxaci Mongolici (*Pu Gong Ying*), 50g, were added.

Complete cure consisted of obvious disappearance of the signs and symptoms with no recurrence within a half year. Based on this criteria, 28 cases or 70% experienced complete cure. Some improvement was defined as obvious diminishment of the signs and symptoms. Eight cases or 20% fell into this category. Only 4 cases or 10% failed to experience any improvement.

Case history: Female, 46 years old. Nine months previously the patient had experienced emotional upset. At that time, she felt something in her throat which she could neither swallow down nor spit up. When eating, her throat was normal and there was no obvious aching or pain. She also experienced abdominal distention and oppression extending to both lateral costal regions. She had tried numerous formulas but without result. Examination revealed that her lips were slightly dry, her urine was yellow, and her stools were dry. Her tongue coating was slightly yellow and her pulse was wiry and slippery. Her pattern was thus categorized as liver depression and qi counterflow, loss of harmony of the spleen and stomach, and phlegm qi counterflowing upward. It was, therefore, appropriate that her treatment mainly consisted of coursing the liver and resolving depression, rectifying the qi and transforming phlegm. The medicinals employed consisted of _Shun Qi Xiao Shi Hua Tan Tang_ plus Cortex Cinnamomi (_Gui Yuan Rou_), 10g, and Fructus Gardeniae Jasminoidis (_Zhi Zi_), 10g. After 3 _ji_, her symptoms had disappeared. After another 5 _ji_, her disease was completely cured. On follow-up after 1 year, there had been no recurrence.

"The Treatment of 54 Cases of Plum Pit Qi with _Bai Mei Li Yan Tang_ (Peony & Mume Disinhibiting the Throat Decoction)" by Zhang Jian-hua, _Shang Hai Zhong Yi Yao Za Zhi (The Shanghai Journal of Traditional Chinese Medicine & Medicinals)_, #1, 1992, p. 20-1; BF

This clinical audit discusses the effects of _Bai Mei Li Yan Tang_ on what is known in the West as neurotic esophageal stenosis or globus hystericus. This formula consists of: Radix Albus Paeoniae Lactiflorae (_Sheng Bai Shao_), 9g, Flos Pruni Mume (_Lu E Mei_), 4.5g, Radix Adenophorae Strictae (_Nan Sha Shen_), 4.5g, Bulbus Lilii (_Chuan Bai He_), 9g, Radix Platycodi Grandiflori (_Bai Jie Gen_), 4.5g, Rhizoma Belamcandae (_She Gan_), 4.5g, and Radix Glycyrrhizae (_Sheng Gan Cao_), 3g.

A number of modifications are given for this formula. Unfortunately, several of them are very unusual ingredients or unusual names for common ingredients the translator has not been able to identify. These are given in Pinyin only. For dizziness and vertigo due to liver hyperactivity, Ramulus Uncariae Cum Uncis (*Diao Teng Gou*), Fructus Tribuli Terrestris (*Bai Ji Li*), etc.were added. For liver qi depression and binding with chest oppression and qi inversion, Tuber Curcumae (*Guang Yu Jin*), Flos Citri Sacrodactylis (*Fo Shou Hua*), *Ye Qiang Wei Hua*, mix-fried Fructus Citri Seu Ponciri (*Chao Zhi Ke*), etc. were added. For heart palpitations and insomnia, Sclerotium Pararadicis Poriae Cocos (*Fu Shen*), Fructus Schizandrae Chinensis (*Wu Wei Zi*), processed Radix Polygalae Tenuifoliae (*Zhi Yuan Zhi*), Flos Albizziae Julibrissinis (*He Huan Hua*), etc. were added. For pasty phlegm in the head of the throat which is not able to be easily spit out, Fructus Arctii (*Niu Bang Zi*), Bulbus Fritillariae Thunbergii (*Bei Mu*), *Di Ku Luo*, etc. were added. For yin vacuity dry throat with scant fluids, Radix Trichosanthis Kirlowii (*Tian Hua Fen*), Radix Scrophulariae Ningpoensis (*Bei Yuan Shen*), etc. were added. And for spleen vacuity with damp accumulation and torpid intake, Radix Glycyrrhizae was deleted and parched Rhizoma Atractylodis Macrocephalae (*Jiao Bia Zhu*), Radix Dioscoreae Oppositae (*Huai Shan Yao*), Massa Medica Fermentata (*Shen Qu*), etc. were added.

One packet of the above ingredients was decocted each day. The resulting liquid was divided in two and these 2 doses were taken per day. Two weeks of such treatment constituted 1 complete course of therapy. Twenty-one or 38.9% of the cases experienced obvious improvement after 2 whole courses of therapy. Another 28 cases or 51.8% experienced some improvement. Five cases experienced no improvement or 9.3%. The total amelioration rate in this study was, therefore, 90.7%.

"The Treatment of 64 Cases of Chronic Laryngitis with *Xue Fu Zhu Yu Tang* (Blood Mansion Dispelling Stasis Decoction)" by Li Xin-cun, *Bei Jing Zhong Yi (Beijing Traditional Chinese Medicine)*, #6, 1993, p. 48; BF

This clinical audit reports on the treatment of 64 cases of chronic inflammation of the throat. The author begins by equating this condition with what is called plum pit qi in Traditional Chinese Medicine. This condition mostly occurs in adults. Of the 64 patients treated with this formula, 23 were men and 41 were women. Thus the male to female ratio was 1:1.8. The youngest patient was 18 years old and the oldest was 54. The shortest disease course was 8 days and the longest was 4 years. The main symptoms of these patients' condition were hyperemia of the throat, dry throat, sore throat, itchy throat, and the feeling as if something were stuck in the throat which spitting could not discharge and swallowing could not descend. Twenty-five cases mainly experienced a dry, sore throat, and 39 mainly experienced an itchy throat and the feeling as if something were stuck in the throat.

Xue Fu Zhu Yu Tang consists of: Radix Angelicae Sinensis (*Dang Gui*), 15g, Flos Carthami Tinctorii (*Hong Hua*), 10g, Semen Pruni Persicae (*Tao Ren*), 10g, Fructus Citri Seu Ponciri (*Zhi Ke*), 10g, Radix Bupleuri (*Chai Hu*), 10g, Radix Rubrus Paeoniae Lactiflorae (*Chi Shao*), 15g, Rhizoma Ligustici Wallichii (*Chuan Xiong*), 10g, Radix Platycodi Grandiflori (*Jie Geng*), 10g, Radix Cyathulae (*Chuan Niu Xi*), 15g, raw Radix Rehmanniae (*Sheng Di*), 15g, and Radix Glycyrrhizae (*Gan Cao*), 10g. These were decocted in water and administered, 1 *ji* per day.

If there was a dry, sore throat, Radix Scrophulariae Ningpoensis (*Yuan Shen*), 15g, Radix Trichosanthis Kirlowii (*Hua Fen*), 15g, and mix-fried Folium Eriobotryae Japonicae (*Zhi Ba Ye*), 10g, were added. If there was itchy throat, Rhizoma Belamcandae (*She Gan*), 10g, and Herba Menthae (*Bo He*), 10g, were added. If there was the feeling as if something were stuck in the throat, Caulis Perillae Frutescentis (*Su Geng*), 10g, and Rhizoma Pinelliae Ternatae (*Ban Xia*), 10g, were added. Ten *ji* equalled 1 course of treatment.

41

Complete cure consisted of the disappearance of the clinical symptoms and no hyperemia of the throat, and marked improvement consisted of diminishment of the clinical symptoms. Based on these criteria, 52 cases or 81.2% were cured, 11 or 17.2% experienced marked improvement, and only 1 or 1.6% experienced no result. Thus the total amelioration rate was 98.4%. The smallest number of *ji* administered was 8 and the largest was 20, the average being 14.

Case history: Female, 28 years old. The patient had felt like she had something stuck in her throat for 3 years. This could neither be spit up nor swallowed down. In addition, her throat was dry and sometimes itchy. She also experienced vexation and agitation. She had been treated previously with Western medical anti-inflammatories but without success. When she came for examination, her throat was hyperemic, her tongue was dark red with static spots on its edges and a thin, white coating, and her pulse was deep and wiry. Treatment consisted of quickening the blood and transforming stasis, resolving depression and disinhibiting the throat.

For this, *Xue Fu Zhu Yu Tang* with additions and subtractions was employed: Radix Angelicae Sinensis (*Dang Gui*), 15g, Flos Carthami Tinctorii (*Hong Hua*), 10g, Semen Pruni Persicae (*Tao Ren*), 10g, Fructus Citri Seu Ponciri (*Zhi Ke*), 10g, Radix Bupleuri (*Chai Hu*), 10g, Radix Rubrus Paeoniae Lactiflorae (*Chi Shao*), 15g, raw Radix Rehmanniae (*Sheng Di*), 20g, Radix Platycodi Grandiflori (*Jie Geng*), 10g, Radix Cyathulae (*Chuan Niu Xi*), 15g, Radix Glycyrrhizae (*Gan Cao*), 6g, Caulis Perillae Frutescentis (*Su Geng*), 10g, Rhizoma Pinelliae Ternatae (*Ban Xia*), 10g, and Radix Scrophulariae Ningpoensis (*Yuan Shen*), 15g. These were decocted in water and administered, 1 *ji* per day.

After taking 6 *ji*, the hyperemia had disappeared and the dry throat, occasional itching, and the feeling as if something were stuck in the throat had diminished. Therefore, Scrophularia was subtracted from the above formula and Cortex Magnoliae Officinalis (*Chuan Po*), 10g, was added. Administration was stopped after she was given another 5 *ji*. At that point, all her symptoms had disappeared and, on follow-up a half year later, there had been no recurrence.

Rheumatoid Arthritis

"The Treatment of 27 Cases of Rheumatoid Arthritis with *She Cong San* (Snake & Insect Powder)" by Shi Qing-pei, *Jiang Su Zhong Yi (Jiangsu Traditional Chinese Medicine)*, #2, 1993, p. 17-8; BF

This clinical audit describes the treatment of 27 patients suffering from rheumatoid arthritis. Twenty-five of these patients were women and 2 were men. They ranged in age from 15-57 years with most falling between 21-37 years of age. The course of their disease had lasted from 4 months to 19 years. Treatment consisted of three parts. First, everyone in this study received the same herbal capsules. Secondly, patients were administered patent medicines based on pattern discrimination. And third, patients were given either of two herbal soaks, one for those who were predominately cold and the other for those who were predominately hot.

She Cong San: Agkistrodon Seu Bungarus (*Bai Hua She*), 10 strips, processed Scolopendra Subspinipes (*Zhi Wu Gong*), 20 strips, processed Buthus Martensis (*Zhi Quan Xie*), 30g, processed Nidus Vespae (*Zhi Feng Fang*), Lumbricus (*Guang Di Long*) and Bombyx Batryticatus (*Bai Jiang Can*), 100g @, and processed Semen Strychnotis (*Zhi Ma Qian Zi*), 20g.

The Semen Strychnotis was first boiled with Semen Phaseoli Munginis (*Lu Dou*). The Semen Strychnotis was then removed and their skins taken off. They were cut into slices and fried in earth until they turned brown. The other six ingredients should be baked slowly over a fire until dry. Then all the ingredients were ground together into a fine powder. The resulting powder was packed into "0" sized capsules till they weighed about 900-1000 mg per capsule. Eight such capsules were taken 3 times per day. Forty days comprised 1 course of therapy.

Chinese Patent Medicines prescribed on the Basis of Pattern Discrimination

There were 6 cases of wind cold dampness pattern who received *Mu Gua Wan* (Chaenomelis Pills), 15 pills 3 times per day. One patient with wind damp heat pattern received *San Miao Wan* (Three Wonders Pills), 6g 3 times per day. Eight patients with phlegm stasis mutually obstructing received *Xiao Huo Luo Wan* (Small Quicken the Connecting Vessels Pills), 1 pill 2 times per day. Two cases of qi and blood insufficiency received *Bu Zhong Yi Qi Wan* (Supplement the Center, Boost the Qi Pills), 6g 3 times per day, or *Shi Quan Da Bu Gao* (Ten Complete Great Supplementing Paste), 15g 3 times per day. Three cases of decline of *ming men* fire were given *Quan Lu Wan* (Whole Deer Pills), 6g 2 times per day. Two cases with liver/kidney yin vacuity pattern were administered *Liu Wei Di Huang Wan* (Six Flavor Rehmannia Pills), 8 pills 3 times per day. And 5 patients with yin vacuity, fire effulgent were given *Zhi Bai Di Huang Wan* (Anemarrhena & Phellodendron Rehmannia Pills), 8 pills 3 times per day.

Fumigation/Wash Formula: Herba Cum Radice Asari Sieboldi (*Xi Xin*), 20g, Radix Clematidis (*Wei Ling Xian*), 15g, Cortex Erythrinae (*Hai Dong Pi*), Fructus Liquidambaris Taiwaniae (*Lu Lu Tong*), Spina Gleditschiae Chinensis (*Zao Jiao Ci*), Herba Tougucao (*Tou Gu Cao*), Cortex Radicis Acanthopanacis (*Wu Jia Pi*), Lumbricus (*Di Long*), and Radix Kaempferiae Galangae (*Shan Nai*), 10g @. If cold was more serious, raw Radix Aconiti (*Sheng Chuan Wu*), raw Radix Aconiti (*Sheng Cao Wu*), and Ramulus Cinnamomi (*Gui Zhi*), 10g @, were added. If heat was more serious, Caulis Lonicerae Japonicae (*Ren Dong Teng*) and raw Radix Et Rhizoma Rhei (*Sheng Da Huang*), 15g

@, were added. This was decocted in 5000 ml of water and boiled for 5 minutes. Then alcohol (*Bai Jiu*) and vinegar (*Shi Cu*), 50g @, were added. While hot, the liquid was used to fumigate and wash the affected joints. One *ji* or packet of the above medicinals can be used for 2 days. Each day, this treatment was done 2 times for 1 hour each time.

Of the 27 cases treated with the above combined protocol, only 1 (3.7%) was completely cured. Nine (33.3%) experienced marked improvement. Another 14 (51.9%) experienced some improvement, and 3 (11.1%) experienced no result. Thus the overall amelioration rate was 88.9%. However, several patients did experience some side effects from the *She Chong San*. Three patients suffered from loss of appetite and nausea, one from generalized pruritus, and one from dizziness. Dr. Shi mentions that if a patient exhibits two patterns simultaneously, such as wind cold dampness and qi and blood insufficiency, they should be given both appropriate Chinese patent medicines.

Heel Pain

"The Treatment of 84 Cases of Heel Pain Employing Measures for Boosting the Qi & Transforming Stasis" by Xie Ke-shui, *Shang Hai Zhong Yi Yao Za Zhi (The Shanghai Journal of Traditional Chinese Medicine & Medicinals)*, #5, 1992, p. 18; CC

Of the 84 cases in this study, 38 were male and 46 were female. Forty experienced left heel pain, and 44 experienced right heel pain. There were 49 patients between the ages of 40-60 and 35 patients between the ages of 61-80 years old. There were 61 patients whose course of illness ranged from 3-12 months and 23 patients whose illness had lasted more than 12 months. Thirty-one patients were diagnosed with heel spurs via x-ray, 17 of which were on the left heel and 14 of which were on the right heel. Patients were divided into two types based upon the nature of the heel pain. Type I (46-cases): When at rest there was no obvious pain and soreness, while there was pain and soreness with walking. Type II (38-cases): There was pain and soreness while both at rest and walking.

The patients took nothing but *Yi Qi Hua Yu Tang* (Boosting Qi, Transforming Stasis Decoction) during their course of therapy. This consisted of the following ingredients: Radix Astragali Membranacei (*Huang Qi*), 20g, Radix Angelicae Sinensis (*Dang Gui*), 12g, Radix Salviae Miltiorrhizae (*Dan Shen*), 15g, Radix Ligustici Wallichii (*Chuan Xiong*), 12g, Radix Rubrus Paeoniae Lactiflorae (*Chi Shao*), 12g, Radix Achyranthis Bidentatae (*Niu Xi*), 15g, and Rhizoma Corydalis Yanhusuo (*Yuan Hu*), 15g. One *ji* was decocted each day and administered twice daily. Fourteen to 21 days constituted one course of treatment.

Fifty-three cases achieved an excellent therapeutic effect. This was defined as a complete disappearance of pain while walking and at rest. Twenty-eight cases achieved a good therapeutic effect. This was defined as disappearance of pain while resting and a lessening of pain while walking. The total of these two groups reflected an 85.7% success rate.

"Chinese Medicinal Therapy in the Treatment of Painful Heels: A Clinical Analysis of 207 Cases" by Wu Ya-ping, *Zhong Guo Zhong Yi Shang Gu Ke Za Zhi (The Chinese Journal of Traditional Chinese Medicine Traumatology & Orthopedics)*, #5, 1991, p. 34; CC

This study reports on the clinical efficacy of both internally administered and externally applied Chinese medicinals for the treatment of heel pain. Treatment was given based on a discrimination of patterns.

1. Kidney vacuity pattern (26 cases)

The treatment principles for this pattern were to supplement the kidneys and strengthen the yang.

Topical medication consisted of: Herba Epimedii (*Xian Ling Pi*), 30g, Radix Astragali Membranacei (*Huang Qi*), 30g, Rhizoma Gusuibu (*Gu Sui Bu*), 30g, Caulis Millettiae Seu Spatholobi (*Ji Xue Teng*), 30g, Herba Cum Radice Asari Sieboldi (*Xi Xin*), 20g, Radix Ledebouriellae Sesloidis (*Fang Feng*), 20g, Radix Praeparatus Aconiti Carmichaeli (*Fu Zi*), 20g, Spina Gleditschiae Chinensis (*Zao Jiao Ci*), 20g, Rhizoma Arisaematis (*Nan Xing*), 10g, Rhizoma Pinelliae Ternatae (*Ban Xia*), 10g, Radix Aconiti (*Chuan Wu*), 10g, and Radix Aconiti (*Cao Wu*), 10g.

Internal medication consisted of: Herba Epimedii (*Xian Ling Pi*), 40g, Radix Astragali Membranacei (*Huang Qi*), 40g, Rhizoma Gusuibu (*Gu Sui Bu*), 30g, Caulis Millettiae Seu Spatholobi (*Ji Xue Teng*), 30g, Radix Ledebouriellae Sesloidis (*Fang Feng*), 20g, Radix Rubrus Paeoniae Lactiflorae (*Chi Shao*), 15g, Radix Albus Paeoniae Lactiflorae (*Bai Shao*), 15g, Radix Aconiti (*Bai Fu Zi*), 15g (precook), Spina Gleditschiae Chinensis (*Zao Jiao Ci*), 10g, and Ramulus Cinnamomi (*Gui Zhi*), 6g.

2. Taxation detriment, cold damp pattern (18 cases)

The treatment principles for this pattern were to supplement and boost the qi and blood, disperse cold and strengthen the sinews.

Topical medication consisted of: Radix Astragali Membranacei (*Huang Qi*), 30g, Caulis Millettiae Seu Spatholobi (*Ji Xue Teng*), 30g, Radix Praeparatus Aconiti Carmichaeli (*Bai Fu Zi*), 30g, Radix Dipsaci (*Xu Duan*), 15g, Eupolyphaga Seu Opisthoplatia (*Di Bie Chong*), 15g, Radix Ledebouriellae Sesloidis (*Fang Feng*), 10g, Spina Gleditschiae

Chinensis (*Zao Jiao Ci*), 10g, Herba Cum Radice Asari Sieboldi (*Xi Xin*), 10g, Radix Aconiti (*Chuan Wu*), 10g, Radix Aconiti (*Cao Wu*), 10g, Gummum Olibani (*Ru Xiang*), 6g, and Myrrha (*Mo Yao*), 6g.

Internal medication consisted of: Caulis Millettiae Seu Spatholobi (*Ji Xue Teng*), 30g, Radix Astragali Membranacei (*Huang Qi*), 30g, Radix Ledebouriellae Sesloidis (*Fang Feng*), 15g, Radix Dipsaci (*Xu Duan*), 15, Radix Rubrus Paeoniae Lactiflorae (*Chi Shao*), 15g, Radix Albus Paeoniae Lactiflorae (*Bai Shao*), 15g, Radix Praeparatus Aconiti Carmichaeli (*Bai Fu Zi*), 15g (precook), Eupolyphaga Seu Opistho-platia (*Di Bie Chong*), 10g, Spina Gleditschiae Chinensis (*Zao Jiao Ci*), 10g, and Ramulus Cinnamomi (*Gui Zhi*), 6g.

3. Blood stasis due to injury pattern (9 cases)

The treatment principles for this pattern were to quicken the blood and transform stasis, unblock the connecting vessels and arrest pain.

Topical medication consisted of: Semen Pruni Persicae (*Tao Ren*), 20g, Flos Carthami Tinctorii (*Hong Hua*), 20g, Semen Vaccariae Segetalis (*Wang Bu Liu Xing*), 20g, Caulis Akebiae Mutong (*Mu Tong*), 20g, Spina Gleditschiae Chinensis (*Zao Jiao Ci*), 15g, Radix Aconiti (*Chuan Wu*), 15g, Radix Aconiti (*Cao Wu*), 15g, Rhizoma Arisaematis (*Nan Xing*), 15g, Rhizoma Pinelliae Ternatae (*Ban Xia*), 15g, Radix Sophorae Subprostratae (*Shan Dou Gen)*, 15g, Rhizoma Ligustici Wallichii (*Chuan Xiong*), 10g, Ramulus Cinnamomi (*Gui Zhi*), 10g, and Rhizoma Atractylodis (*Cang Zhu*), 10g.

Internal medication: none

Methods of preparation and application:

Topical medication: Each of the ingredients in the prescription were dried and powdered finely. In patterns 1 and 2 above and patients with pattern 3 whose illness was more than 3 days old, the ingredients were mixed with boiled water and applied warm to the affected area. A hot water bottle was then placed on the hot plaster. For patients with pattern 3 whose illness was less than 3 days old, the ingredients were mixed with cold water and applied cold to the affected area. Regardless of whether the medicinals were applied cold or warm, they were applied for a duration of time ranging from 30 minutes to 3 hours, once or twice daily. Each poultice was used 2-3 times. In addition, in patterns 1 and 2 and in patients with pattern 3 whose illness was more than 3 days old, the dregs from both the internal and topical therapies (the topical paste having been wrapped in a cloth bag) were added to boiling water. The affected area was first fumigated and then soaked for 20 minutes once or twice daily. At the same time, light massage was applied to the affected area. The dregs from the fumigation and soak were reused 1-2 times. Whereas the fresh ingredients from the internal medication were used 3-4 times. The above two techniques were either combined or used singly.

Internal medication: The medicinals for internal medication were decocted for 15 minutes and were administered to patients with patterns 1 and 2 for whom topical medication had shown no obvious effect or who complained of accompanying low back and knee soreness and weakness and lack of strength. One *ji* was administered over 2 days, 3-4 times per day. These therapies were not used on patients presenting with obvious inflammation or broken skin. If, following administration of the paste, the skin became excessively irritated, this method was suspended.

Complete cure consisted of a disappearance of heel pain and normalizing of function. Positive result consisted of a basic disappearance of heel pain and a basic recovery of function. No result was defined as a persistence of heel pain, impairment of function, and no obvious changes when compared to the condition before therapy. The least number of topical and internal *ji* required was 1, the greatest was 9. The shortest duration of therapy was 3 days and the longest was 20 days. Based on the above criteria, 38 cases experienced a complete cure, 12 cases experienced a positive result, and 3 cases experienced no result. Ninety-two point thirty-one percent of those with the kidney vacuity pattern were treated successfully, 94.45% of those with the taxation detriment damp cold pattern were treated successfully, and 100% of those with blood stasis due to injury were treated successfully.

Redness & Pain of the Extremities

"The Treatment of 42 Cases of Redness & Pain in the Extremities Using *Ma Xing Gan Shi Tang* (Ephedra, Armeniaca, Licorice & Gypsum Decoction) with Additions" by Niu Zhi-shi, *Bei Jing Zhong Yi Xue Yuan Za Zhi (The Beijing College of Traditional Chinese Medicine Journal)*, #5, 1993, p. 51; CC

Redness and pain in the extremities are characterized by a localized increase in the temperature of the extremities due to a periodic dilation of the blood vessels. Forty-two cases of this disease were treated with *Ma Xing Gan Shi Tang* with satisfactory results. Of the 42 participants in this study, 39 were male and 3 were female. They ranged in age from 15-35 years of age with the median age being 25 years old. The course of the illness ranged from one month to 5 years with the median duration being 28 months. The etiology of the illness was attributed to an exposure to high temperatures in 17 cases, to freezing in 13 cases, to infection in 5 cases, and to unknown causes in 7 cases. All 42 cases had the symptoms in both lower extremities.

The characteristic symptoms included an acute onset of burning in both legs and severe stabbing pain, both of which were episodic in nature. The temperature of the skin was elevated and had a reddish cast, and the symptoms were diminished when both legs were immersed in cold water. The tongue coating was typically red with a dry, white or yellow coating. The pulse was typically wiry and rapid or slippery and rapid.

Diagnostic criteria were based on *Shi Yong Zhong Xi Jie He Zhen Duan Zhi Liao Xue (Commonly Used Integrated Chinese-Western Diagnoses & Therapies)*, July, 1991 edition: There was severe pain when the extremities were exposed to heat. When the symptoms were present, they could be ameliorated or would disappear altogether when the lower limb was cooled in some way. There was an increase in the strength of the surrounding pulses and a corresponding increase in surrounding blood flow in those blood vessels.

The prescription contained: Herba Ephedrae (*Ma Huang*), 9-20g, Gypsum (*Shi Gao*), 15-200g, stir-fried Semen Pruni Armeniacae (*Xing Ren*), 9g, Periostracum Cicadae (*Chan Tui*), 30-60g, Lumbricus (*Di Long*), 15-30g, and Radix Glycyrrhizae (*Gan Cao*), 9-30g. If the toes were especially red, swollen, hot, and painful and the symptoms were continuous, then Cornu Bubali (*Shui Niu Jiao*), 12-30g, Rhizoma Anemarrhenae (*Zhi Mu*), 15g, and Cortex Radicis Moutan (*Dan Pi*), 12g, were added to the prescription. One *ji* was administered daily. The first 2 decoctions were divided into 2 doses and administered orally. A third decoction was applied as a fomentation to both legs, twice daily for a period of about 30 minutes at a temperature of between 20-28 C. Patients were prohibited from smoking, drinking (alcohol), or eating spicy foods.

Therapeutic criteria were also based on *Commonly Used Integrated Chinese-Western Diagnoses & Therapies*: If the patient was no longer in pain and exposure to heat no longer triggered the illness, this was defined as a complete cure. If the patient experienced fewer episodes or a complete disappearance of pain but exposure to heat still triggered the illness, this was defined as positive changes. The therapy was considered ineffective if the pain and soreness remained, was still periodic in nature, and continued to be triggered by exposure to heat.

Of the 42 cases studied, 34 achieved a clinical cure, and 8 obtained a positive result, yielding an overall amelioration rate of 89%. The course of therapy lasted from 15-45 days, with the average being 19 days.

Redness and pain of the extremities falls within the scope of heat *bi* in Chinese medicine. This is most commonly due to the contraction of a heat pathogen or a cold pathogen which becomes internally depressed and transforms into heat. This heat pathogen depresses the striae and obstructs the channels and connecting vessels. In using the treatment measure of "effusing depressive fire", the author employed acrid, dissipating, diffusing, and out-thrusting medicinals to provide the pathogen with an exit. Once the pathogen had left the skin, the condition was cured. In this prescription, Ephedra regulates the blood vessels and diffuses and dissipates the depressive pathogen from the level of the skin. This is supported by Gypsum and Periostracum Cicadae which clear and dissipate depressive heat. Armeniaca circulates the depressed and stagnant qi, Lumbricus transforms stagnant heat and unblocks the channels and connecting vessels, and raw Licorice clears heat and drains fire as well as harmonizes the influence of the other medicinals. Pharmacological research has shown that Ephedra, Gypsum, Periostracum Cicadae, Lumbricus, and Licorice all have anti-inflammatory, anti-allergenic, and vasoconstrictive properties. Ephedra, in particular, has been shown to regulate vascular function and is a reliable vasoconstrictor.

To ensure against a relapse of the illness, patients were instructed to continue taking the medication for at least a fortnight after the symptoms had completely disappeared. They were also instructed to avoid strenuous exercise.

Insomnia

"A Comparative Study on the Treatment of Insomnia" by Mo Tai-an, _Jiang Su Zhong Yi (Jiangsu Traditional Chinese Medicine)_, #2, 1993, p. 13; BF

This research report describes a comparative study on the treatment of insomnia. There were 68 patients altogether in this study. Of these, 42 were male and 26 female. Their ages ranged from 16-65 with most patients falling between 30-40 years of age. The duration of their disease went from 1/2 month to 8 years. Typically, the patients complained of insomnia, excessive dreams, heart vexation, poor memory, exhaustion and fatigue, tenseness, agitation, and easy anger, dizziness, heart palpitations, etc.

The patients were divided into two groups. One group was treated with a Chinese herbal formula called _Shu Gan Xie Huo An Shen Tang_ (Course the Liver, Discharge Fire, and Quiet the Spirit Decoction). This group was known as the treatment group. It consisted of 41 patients. The other group, known as the control group, was treated with 20mg 3 times per day of a multivitamin, 20mg 3 times per day of vitamin B_6, and 2.5mg of Valium (_An Ding_) per day given in the evening before bed. One week equalled 1 course of therapy for both groups.

Shu Gan Xie Huo An Shen Tang consists of: Cortex Radicis Moutan (_Dan Pi_), Fructus Gardeniae Jasminoidis (_Zhi Zi_), and Cortex Albizziae Julibrissinis (_He Huan Pi_), 10g @, stir-fried Fructus Zizyphi Spinosae (_Chao Zao Ren_) and Caulis Polygoni Multiflori (_Ye Jiao Teng_), 24g @, Radix Bupleuri (_Chai Hu_), 5g, and Raw Os Draconis (_Sheng Long Gu_) and Raw Conchae Ostreae (_Sheng Mu Li_), 30g @.

If there was parched mouth and dry throat, Radix Glehniae Littoralis (_Sha Shen_) and Tuber Ophiopogonis Japonicae (_Mai Dong_), 15g @, were added. If there was insufficiency of heart qi and blood, Radix Astragali Membranacei (*Huang Qi*) and Arillus Euphoriae Longanae (*Gui Yuan Rou*), 15g @, were added. If there was lack of communication between the heart and kidneys, *Jiao Tai Wan* (Grand Communication Pills) were added. One *ji* was used per day and decocted twice. The first decoction was taken in the afternoon and the second decoction was taken 1/2 hour before sleep.

The criteria for success in this research were defined as follows: Marked improvement consisted of obvious improvement in the length and quality of sleep and the disappearance of such symptoms as heart vexation, tenseness, agitation, easy anger, etc. Some improvement consisted of some improvement in sleep, heart vexation, tenseness, agitation, easy anger, etc. And no result meant that there was no obvious change in any of these parameters. Among the treatment group, 17 cases (41.4%) experienced marked improvement; 22 (53.7%), some improvement; and 2 (4.9%), no result. Among the control group, 2 cases (7.4%) experienced marked improvement; 9 (33.3%), some improvement; and 16 (59.3%), no result.

Dr. Mo says that in TCM, insomnia may have many causes. Worry and taxation and exhaustion may internally damage the heart and spleen. Yang may not communicate with yin and thus the heart and kidneys lose communication. There may be yin vacuity with effulgent fire with liver yang harassing and moving. Or fierce anger may damage the liver, liver qi becoming depressed and transforming into fire. Thus the *hun* may not be able to be treasured and therefore insomnia arises. In this case, the group of symptoms include insomnia, excessive dreams, exhaustion and fatigue, poor memory, heart vexation, tenseness, agitation, easy anger, etc. In TCM, this type of insomnia is categorized as liver depression transforming into fire, fire harassing the heart spirit, and the spirit not being treasured calmly. Therefore, this formula, taken as a whole, has the ability to course the liver and discharge fire, balance and nourish the heart spirit.

Frightful Sleep

"Experience with *Xue Fu Zhu Yu Tang* (Decoction for Eliminating Stasis from the Blood Mansion) in the Treatment of Frightful Sleep", Hu Ji-ming, *Zhe Jiang Zhong Yi Za Zhi (The Zhejiang Journal of Traditional Chinese Medicine)*, #5, 1993, p. 198; CC

Frightful sleep is characterized by interruptions in the normal course of sleep. During the first phase of sleep, the patient will wake with a scream, sitting bolt upright or falling out of bed. The author has treated this disorder successfully with *Xue Fu Zhu Yu Tang* and a representative case history follows.

A 35 year old female was first examined on July 25, 1989. She reported that she would not be asleep for very long before she would suddenly scream and sit up awake with both eyes open wide. This was accompanied by rough respiration and palpitations and tachycardia. The condition would last 10 minutes and then begin to calm down. She would then go back to sleep and the pattern would recur as often as 10 times per night. When she did return to sleep, she rested uneasily as if she were walking on thin ice. Cardiac and neurological examinations revealed nothing abnormal. She had received many therapies previously, including antidepressant medications. However, nothing could control her condition.

When the patient came to see the author, she was restless and had a bitter taste in her mouth. Her pulse was fine and wiry, while her tongue was pale red with a thin, slimy coating. The patient was given *Xue Fu Zhu Yu Tang* with additions. This contained: 10g each of Radix Angelicae Sinensis (*Dang Gui*), Semen Pruni Persicae (*Tao Ren*), Flos Carthami Tinctorii (*Hong Hua*), Radix Platycodi Grandiflori (*jie Geng*), Radix Rubrus Paeoniae Lactiflorae (*Chi Shao*), Radix Bupleuri (*Chai Hu*), Fructus Immaturus Citri Seu Ponciri (*Zhi Shi*),

Rhizoma Ligustici Wallichi (*Chuan Xiong*), Radix Achyranthis Bidentatae (*Niu Xi*), Rhizoma Pinelliae Ternatae (*Ban Xia*), and Caulis In Taeniis Bambusae (*Dan Zhu Ru*). It also contained: raw Concha Haliotidis (*Sheng Jue Ming*), 30g, Margaritiferae (*Zhen Zhu Mu*), 30g, and Pericarpium Citri Reticulatae (*Chen Pi*), 5g. This was decocted in water and 7 *ji* were administered.

The frequency of the episodes markedly diminished even though she would still wake up suddenly. Nevertheless, she no longer had a frightened expression, her mind became clearer, and she was less obviously anxious. She had some slight soreness and pain in the temporal region, thoracic oppression, vexatious heat in the five hearts, and poor sleep. Her pulse was fine and wiry, and her tongue was red with a thin coating. Therefore, *Dang Gui*, Platycodon, Caulis In Taeniis Bambusae, and Orange Peel were deleted from the original prescription and raw Radix Rehmanniae (*Sheng Di*), 10g, Rhizoma Anemarrhenae (*Zhi Mu*), 10g, Semen Biotae (*Bai Zi Ren*) 10g, and Cortex Phellodendri (*Chuan Bai*), 3g, were added and 7 more *ji* were administered. At this time, the fright ceased altogether. However, the symptoms returned again in April, 1992. A single dose of the same prescription was administered and this arrested the illness and, up to the present day, it has not returned.

According to Dr. Hu, this illness falls within the scope of fright patterns in Chinese medicine. Typically, gallbladder-warming and heart-nourishing measures are most commonly employed. Heavy use of spirit-calming medicinals is also common based upon the axiom, "If there is fright, level it." Nonetheless, these approaches had produced little effect in this case. It states in "The Discourse on the True Statements of the Golden Cabinet (*Jin Gui Zhen Yen Lun*)" in the *Su Wen (Simple Questions)*:

> The green-blue hue of the eastern direction enters and unblocks the liver. It opens the portals to the eyes and is stored with the essence in the liver and causes the illness of fright.

"The Discourse on Extraordinary Things (*Da Qi Lun*)" in the *Ling Shu (Spiritual Pivot)* states, "When there is an accumulation in the liver, there is fullness in both flanks and lying down causes fright."

The classical explanation for this illness is typically based on the statement, "The liver stores the *hun*." The implications of this statement are that a failure of circulation of the qi and blood in the liver itself, failure of the blood to nourish the liver, or a contraction of a pathogen by the liver may all result in a failure of the liver to store the *hun*. In the author's experience, the primary disease mechanism of this illness is a stagnation of qi and blood accompanied by a vacuity of liver blood. The liver itself is yin and utilizes yang. If there is an orderly reaching of the qi and blood of the liver organ, activity and quietude assist one another, yin and yang are in harmony, the blood is effulgent and nourishes the *hun*, and the spirit is intact and the *hun* is stored, then how can there be fright?

Therefore, liver is central to a number of disease mechanisms which may produce fright. First, when the qi dynamic fails to course the qi, there is stagnation of liver blood, and when there is blood vacuity, the liver is not nourished. Thus, the liver may directly cause fright. Secondly, the liver has an interior/exterior relationship with the gallbladder. When the liver qi becomes stagnant, this impairs the gallbladder's capacity for coursing and draining. When there is an insufficiency of liver blood, this often causes an insufficiency of gallbladder qi resulting in fright. Third, there is an intimate connection between the heart and the liver. If there is either a debility or stagnation of liver qi and blood, then the qi and blood cannot ascend to nourish the heart. The spirit is not nourished and protected, resulting in palpitation fright. This is a case of an illness of the mother affecting the son. Fourth, if the liver fails to course and drain the qi and the qi dynamic malfunctions, this causes a loss of proper ascension and descension allowing the liver qi to attack the lungs. Once the lungs lose their function of diffusion and downbearing, this produces difficult respiration, thoracic oppression or pain, and a sense of precordial pressure.

Xue Fu Zhu Yu Tang was composed by Wang Qing-ren in the Qing dynasty. In his *Yi Lin Gao Cuo (Correction of the Errors of the Medical Forest)*, he states: "When there is nocturnal restlessness....with throbbing heart and flusteredness, and when *Gui Pi* (Returning the Spleen [Decoction]) has proven effective, this prescription (*i.e., Xue Fu Zhu Yu Tang*) hits the mark one hundred times in one hundred." In this prescription, raw Rehmannia, *Dang Gui*, Persica, Carthamus, Red Peony, and Ligusticum to quicken and cool the blood and nourish the blood and yin. Bupleurum, Citrus Immaturus, Red Peony, and Licorice are Zhang Zhong-jing's *Si Ni San* (Four Counterflows Powder) which enters the liver channel and soothes the qi dynamic of the liver and gallbladder. Platycodon opens the lung qi and smoothes the upper warmer, and Achyranthes guides the blood downward, encouraging the blood stasis to drain from the liver. When these medicinals are all combined, qi and blood are addressed equally, and attack and supplementation are administered simultaneously. This allows the *hun* to return to the liver and the heart to store the spirit. The gallbladder qi flows, ascension and descension are uninhibited, and fright is cured.

The author has found this prescription quite effective given an appropriate diagnosis. Typically, only 5 *ji* are necessary to produce a positive result. The additions of raw Abalone Shell and Mother of Pearl enhance the results. If the tongue coating is white and slimy, one may add Pinellia and Orange Peel. If there is vexatious heat in the five hearts, one may add Anemarrhena and Phellodendron. When one tends to awake from sleep easily, Semen Biotae and Salvia may be added.

Spontaneous Perspiration

"The Treatment of Spontaneous Perspiration Using Measures for Quickening the Blood & Transforming Stasis" by Chen Hua-zhang, *Zhong Yi Za Zhi (The Journal of Traditional Chinese Medicine)*, #10, 1993, p. 633; CC

The author notes that the use of measures for quickening the blood and transforming stasis as a means of treating spontaneous perspiration is not often discussed in the medical literature. They then present a representative case employing *Xue Fu Zhu Yu Tang* (Decoction for Eliminating Stasis from the Blood Mansion) in the treatment of this disorder.

A 35 year old textile worker was first examined on June 28, 1984. Four months previously, she had undergone sterilization surgery and since then she had become depressed and was rarely happy. She experienced thoracic oppression and sighing, lack of appetite, headache, insomnia, and tension in her extremities. In the past 2 months, she had developed a sense of thoracic oppression as if there were an obstruction in her chest, and, for the last 10 days, her head had been perspiring. This perspiration had become oily and she would soak her clothing 5-6 times per day, although the sweating was relatively mild in the evening. She had a great thirst that neither cold nor hot liquids could quench and a lack of warmth and numbness in her four extremities. Her condition was diagnosed as a neurological disorder by Western medical practitioners and was given atropine. This would sometimes ameliorate the perspiration. She had also taken *Gui Zhi Jia Long Gu Mu Li Tang* (Cinnamon Twig Plus Dragon bone & Oyster Shell Decoction), *Yu Ping Feng San* (Jade Windscreen Powder), and *Shen Fu Tang* (Ginseng & Aconite Decoction) without effect.

She was, therefore, referred to the author for treatment. The patient reported sudden drenching perspiration, 5 or 6 times per day, which would leave her clothing soaked. Following this, a fine perspiration would persist. She was anxious and would heave great sighs. She suffered from thoracic oppression as if there were an obstruction in her chest. And she had cold and damp limbs, pain and distension in the lower abdomen, and amenorrhea. Her tongue had petechiae and a thin, white, dry coating, while her pulse was wiry. This was a pattern of depressive binding of liver qi disrupting the qi dynamic and blood stasis in the chest impeding the transmission of fluids and humors. The treatment plan was to quicken the blood and circulate the qi, course the liver and resolve depression, diffuse and soothe the lung vessels, and secure the exterior and arrest perspiration. Therefore, _Xue Fu Zhu Yu Tang_ was administered.

The prescription contained: Radix Bupleuri (_Chai Hu_), 10g, Radix Rubrus Paeoniae Lactiflorae (_Chi Shao_), 10g, Semen Pruni Persicae (_Tao Ren_), 10g, Flos Carthami Tinctorii (_Hong Hua_) 6g, Lumbricus (_Di Long_) 10g, Radix Angelicae Sinensis (_Dang Gui_), 12g, Rhizoma Ligustici Wallichi (_Chuan Xiong_), 10g, Radix Platycodi Grandiflori (_Jie Geng_), 10g, Fructus Citri Seu Ponciri (_Zhi Ke_), Radix Cyathulae (_Chuan Niu Xi_), 15g, and calcined Concha Ostreae & Os Draconis (_Duan Long Mu_), 30g @ (precooked).

With administration of 3 _ji_, the heavy sweating ceased, although the fine perspiration would occur occasionally. All the other symptoms diminished. The patient was then given 6 _ji_ of _Xiao Yao San_ (Rambling Powder) and _Tao Hong Si Wu Tang_ (Persica & Carthamus Four Materials Decoction) with modifications (unspecified). She began menstruating again and she was cured.

According to Dr. Chen, spontaneous sweating is most often due to a disharmony of the defensive and constructive, qi vacuity causing insecurity, or an internal compression of a heat pathogen. Wang Qing-ren discusses the use of _Xue Fu Zhu Yu Tang_ in the section on "Daytime Perspiration (_Bai Tian Han Chu_)" in his _Yi Lin Gao Cuo (Corrections of the Errors of the Medical Forest)_. He attributes this illness to a depressive restraint damaging the liver and a stagnation of qi and blood. "The

Discourse on Regulating the Menses (*Tiao Jing Lun Pian*)" in the *Su Wen* (*Simple Questions*) states:

> The pathways of the five viscera all emerge along the channels to circulate blood and qi. Hundreds of illnesses are transformed and engendered when there is a disharmony of blood and qi. Therefore, one must protect the channels.

Spontaneous perspiration may result when the channels and connecting vessels become blocked. The liver rules coursing and drainage, while the lungs rule diffusion and effusion. When both are coordinated, they accomplish the task of transforming fluids and humors into perspiration and eliminating them from the body. If the liver becomes depressed or a longstanding illness enters the connecting vessels, then qi and blood may become disharmonious, causing stagnation in the chest. This disrupts the lungs and hence the fluids and humors are not spread along the channels. Therefore, they spill out of the vessels as perspiration. Quickening the blood and transforming stagnation, coursing the liver and rectifying the qi, and promoting free flow in the channels and vessels "protects the channels" as a means of effectively treating perspiration.

Fu Ke
Gynecology _____

Menstrual Disease

"The Treatment of Menstrual Disease with *Hua Gan Jian* (Transform the Liver Decoction) by Wang Cui-ping, *Tian Jin Zhong Yi (Tianjin Traditional Chinese Medicine)*, #2, 1993, p. 8; BF

The author of this article reports on the treatment of various menstrual diseases using *Hua Gan Jian*. This formula is found in Zhang Jie-bin's *Jing Yue Quan Shu (The Complete Writings of [Zhang] Jing-yue)*. It is comprised of: Pericarpium Viridis Citri Reticulatae (*Qing Pi*), Pericarpium Citri Reticulatae (*Chen Pi*), Fructus Gardeniae Jasminoidis (*Zhi Zi*), Cortex Radicis Moutan (*Dan Pi*), Rhizoma Alismatis (*Ze Xie*), Radix Albus Paeoniae Lactiflorae (*Bai Shao*), and Tuber Bolbostemmae Paniculati (*Tu Bei Mu*). This formula is used to treat angry qi damaging the liver with qi counterflow stirring fire resulting in vexatious heat, lateral costal pain, distention, and fullness, stirring blood, etc. This formula resolves liver qi depression, levels qi counterflow, and scatters depressive fire. With various additions and subtractions, it may be used to treat various menstrual diseases.

Early menstruation

Case history: Female 36 years old, married, peasant. For the previous 4 months, this woman's periods had been coming approximately 10 days early. When severe, she would have 2 periods in a single month. The color of the menstruate was purplish red and its amount was excessive. Before the period, she experienced chest oppression,

63

vexation and agitation, and bilateral breast distention and pain. After the period, she suffered from heart palpitations, vertigo, dry mouth, excessive dreams, shortness of breath, fatigue, and low back and knee soreness and weakness. Her tongue was pale with a thin, yellow coating. Her pulse was wiry and fine. This pattern is categorized as liver depression and blood heat with loss of nourishment of the *chong* and *ren*. The treatment principles were, therefore, to course the liver and clear heat, level and supplement the qi and blood in order to nourish the *chong* and *ren*.

She was given *Hua Gan Jian Jia Jian* (Transform the Liver Decoction with Additions & Subtractions): Pericarpium Viridis Citri Reticulatae (*Qing Pi*), 10g, Pericarpium Citri Reticulatae (*Chen Pi*), 10g, Fructus Gardeniae Jasminoidis (*Zhi Zi*), 9g, Radix Albus Paeoniae Lactiflorae (*Bai Shao*), 18g, Radix Bupleuri (*Chai Hu*), 9g, Radix Angelicae Sinensis (*Dang Gui*), 12g, Radix Pseudostellariae (*Tai Zi Shen*), 15g, raw Radix Rehmanniae (*Sheng Di*), 12g, Fructus Ligustri Lucidi (*Nu Zhen Zi*), 15g, and Herba Ecliptae Prostratae (*Han Lian Cao*), 30g. Three *ji* were decocted in water and administered. After taking the above medicinals, her condition immediately improved and her menstruation returned to normal after 2 months of treatment.

Erratic menstruation

Case history: Female, 43 years old, worker. For a half year, this woman's period had been coming sometimes early and sometimes late. Along with her period, she experienced lower abdominal distention and pain, her menstruate was dark red, it contained clots, but its amount was moderate. She commonly had excessive vaginal discharge which was yellow in color and pasty in consistency. This was sometimes accompanied by vaginal itching. Her stools were dry and her urination was yellow. The tip of her tongue was red and it had a thin, yellow coating. Her pulse was wiry and a little rapid. This pattern is categorized as liver qi depression and binding with menstrual irregularity. Its treatment methods are to course the liver and resolve depression, clear heat and eliminate dampness.

She was given *Hua Gan Jian Jia Jian*: Pericarpium Viridis Citri Reticulatae (*Qing Pi*), 10g, Pericarpium Citri Reticulatae (*Chen Pi*), 10g, Radix Bupleuri (*Chai Hu*), 9g, Cortex Radicis Moutan (*Dan Pi*), 10g, Fructus Gardeniae Jasminoidis (*Zhi Zi*), 9g, Radix Angelicae Sinensis (*Dang Gui*), 10g, Tuber Curcumae (*Yu Jin*), 10g, Herba Leonuri Heterophylli (*Kun Cao*), 30g, Semen Coicis Lachryma-jobi (*Yi Mi*), 20g, Rhizoma Atractylodis and Atractylodis Macrocephalae (*Cang Bai Zhu*), 10g @, stir-fried Herba Seu Flos Schizonepetae Tenuifoliae (*Chao Jing Jie*), 10g, Semen Plantaginis (*Che Qian Zi*), 10g, Rhizoma Alismatis (*Ze Xie*), 10g, and Radix Glycyrrhizae (*Gan Cao*), 6g. Three *ji* were decocted in water and administered. After taking these medicinals, there was no result; therefore, another 3 *ji* were given and after that the period came with obvious improvement in premenstrual signs and symptoms. This formula was given again for 10 days before each period for 3 whole months and the period came on time both then and subsequently.

Dysmenorrhea

Case history: Female, 20 years old, student. For 2 years, the patient would have 2 days of lower abdominal pain with her period accompanied by low back and lower limb soreness. When the pain was severe, she would also have chills and sweating. The amount of menstruate was normal but contained blood clots. As soon as these clots were discharged, the pain diminished. The patient was typically vexed and easily angered and her sleep was disturbed. Her tongue was red and her pulse was wiry and fine. This pattern is categorized as liver depression and qi stagnation with blood stasis obstructing the menses. The treatment principles are to course the liver and rectify the qi, quicken the blood and transform stasis.

The patient was given *Hua Gan Jian Jia Jian*: Pericarpium Viridis Citri Reticulatae (*Qing Pi*), 10g, Pericarpium Citri Reticulatae (*Chen Pi*), 10g, Radix Albus Paeoniae Lactiflorae (*Bai Shao*), 18g, Radix Bupleuri (*Chai Hu*), 9g, Tuber Bolbostemmae Paniculati (*Tu Bei Mu*), 12g, Herba Leonuri Heterophylli (*Kun Cao*), 30g, Semen Pruni Persicae (*Tao Ren*), 15g, Radix Salviae Miltiorrhizae (*Dan Shen*), 15g, Tuber Curcumae (*Yu Jin*), 12g, and Radix Glycyrrhizae (*Gan Cao*), 6g. Three *ji* were decocted in water and administered. After taking these medicinals, the period came and the lower abdominal pain was diminished and the clots discharged were smaller. Therefore, Persica was removed from the formula and Radix Pseudostellariae (*Tai Zi Shen*), 30g, was added and another 3 *ji* were given. After her period, the patient felt short of breath and with little strength. Therefore, she was given *Ba Zhen Tang Jia Jian* (Eight Pearls Decoction with Additions & Subtractions). For the next 2 cycles, 1 week before her period, she was treated again as above and was completely cured.

Amenorrhea

Case history: Female, 40 years old, worker. This woman had had high blood pressure for 3 years. Beginning 1 year previous, her period had started coming late and she had had amenorrhea for the last 8 months. Her body was weak and deficient and she was fatigued and without strength. Her spirit was emotionally depressed and her chest and lateral costal regions were not comfortable. She did not sleep well and her appetite was diminished. Her blood pressure was 170/110mm-Hg and her head was distended and painful. Her tongue was purple and dark and her pulse was wiry and rapid. This pattern is categorized as liver depression and qi binding with liver yang hyperactive above. The treatment principles are to course the liver and resolve depression, level the liver and subdue yang.

The patient was given *Hua Gan Tang Jia Jian*: Pericarpium Viridis Citri Reticulatae (*Qing Pi*), 10g, Pericarpium Citri Reticulatae (*Chen Pi*), 10g, Fructus Gardeniae Jasminoidis (*Zhi Zi*), 10g, Tuber

Bolbostemmae Paniculati (*Tu Bei Mu*), 12g, Cortex Radicis Moutan (*Dan Pi*), 10g, Rhizoma Gastrodiae Elatae (*Tian Ma*), 20g, raw Concha Haliotidis (*Sheng Shi Jue*), 30g, Ramulus Uncariae Seu Uncis (*Shuang Gou*), 20g, Radix Achyranthis Bidentatae (*Niu Xi*), 12g, Dens Draconis (*Long Chi*), 30g, Radix Bupleuri (*Chai Hu*), 9g, Radix Albus Paeoniae Lactiflorae (*Bai Shao*), 18g, Fructus Corni Officinalis (*Zhu Rou*), 15g, Fructus Ligustri Lucidi (*Nu Zhen Zi*), 12g, Semen Zizyphi Spinosae (*Zao Ren*), 30g, Radix Glycyrrhizae (*Gan Cao*), 10g, Herba Lycopi Lucidi (*Ze Lan*), 15g, Cortex Phellodendri (*Juan Bai*), 15g, and Herba Leonuri Heterophylli (*Kun Cao*), 30g. Three *ji* were decocted in water and administered.

After taking these medicinals, the patient's blood pressure was 150/90mmHg. Semen Pruni Persicae (*Tao Ren*), 10g, was added and another 7 *ji* administered. After another 5 *ji*, she experienced some insidious lower abdominal pain and had a small amount of dark, blackish colored menstrual blood. Two days later, her menses came on in full and her blood pressure was 140/80mmHg. Radix Salviae Miltiorrhizae (*Dan Shen*), 20g, Caulis Millettiae Seu Spatholobi (*Ji Xue Teng*), 30g, and Ramus Loranthi Seu Visci (*Ji Sheng*), 30g, were added to the previous formula for treatment the next month after which the blood pressure returned to normal and the amenorrhea was cured.

The author comments that the liver is the viscus of wind wood. It stores yin blood and is the abode of ministerial fire. In form it is yin but in function it is yang. If the liver becomes depressed and does not course, the qi mechanism becomes shut and does not flow freely. In that case, ministerial fire may not be able to be disseminated and spread about. Thus stirring fire may damage the blood. As Zhang Jing-yue has said, "Qi counterflow stirs fire." In this case, this may also result in blood stasis, water accumulation, damp obstruction, and phlegm gathering diseases. Further, if there is liver depression and qi

67

stagnation, this will affect the functioning of the *chong* and *ren* resulting in the generation of menstrual diseases.

The correct treatment method for liver depression is based on the saying, "Depressed wood should be out-thrust." Therefore, *Hua Gan Jian* uses no other medicinals than those which course and open. Green Orange Peel courses the liver, loosens the chest, and resolves depressive anger. Gardenia clears heat and diffuses depression. Since heat damages yin blood, it is combined with Peony which enters the blood division. Together these two medicinals supplement blood vacuity while draining liver repletion. Moutan is added to clear blood heat and move blood stagnation. When stagnation is removed and heat eliminated, depression is automatically resolved. Alisma drains and percolates dampness and disinhibits water. Thus protecting against dampness stops accumulation of phlegm. Orange Peel rectifies the qi and transforms phlegm, while Bolbostemma Paniculatum down-bears phlegm and opens binding.

Premenstrual Lip Swelling & Pain

"One Case of Premenstrual Swelling & Pain of the Mouth Lips Treated by *Xie Huang San* (Draining Yellow Powder)" by Zhang Shu-min, *Bei Jing Zhong Yi (Beijing Traditional Chinese Medicine)*, #6, 1993, p. 46; BF

Xie Huang San originally comes from the *Xiao Er Yao Zheng Zhi Jue (Proven, Straightforward Rhymes [Concerning] Medicinals for Children)*. It was meant to treat pediatric spleen heat affecting the tongue. The fifth edition of *Fang Ji Xue (The Study of Formulas & Prescriptions)* says it is also able to treat spleen/stomach hidden heat, oral ulcers, bad breath, vexatious thirst, easy hunger, a dry mouth and lips, etc. Composed of Herba Agastachis Seu Pogostemi (*Huo Xiang Ye*), Fructus Gardeniae Jasminoidis (*Shan Zhi Zi*), Gypsum (*Shi Gao*),

Radix Glycyrrhizae (*Gan Cao*), and Radix Ledebouriellae Sesloidis (*Fang Feng*), this formula is capable of draining spleen/stomach hidden fire.

Case history: Female, 42 years old, cadre. This woman came for her first diagnosis in November, 1988. For one year previously, each time before her period came, her lips would become swollen and painful. She had already been treated with Western medical antibiotics and vitamins, but with no obvious improvement. Therefore, she had come for TCM diagnosis and treatment. Her condition manifested as swollen and enlarged lips of the mouth. Her lips were red and when she ate, her lips would crack causing extreme aching and pain. The mucosa inside her oral cavity was normal, and after the period, her condition relaxed and resolved. The amount of her menstrual blood was categorized as excessive. Its color was dark and contained clots. Her period lasted 7-8 days. Her last period had come on Oct. 22. This month her period had not yet come. Abnormal vaginal discharge was colored yellow but was not excessive in amount. For the last half day, her stools had been dry and knotted. She was vexed, tense, and easily angered. Her tongue was pale red with a yellow coating, and her pulse was wiry and rapid.

Her pattern discrimination was spleen/stomach stagnant heat which flamed upward with the period. The treatment principles were to drain heat and scatter fire, cool the blood and regulate the menses. The formula consisted of: Herba Agastachis Seu Pogostemi (*Huo Xiang*), 20g, Fructus Gardeniae Jasminoidis (*Shan Zhi Zi*), 10g, Gypsum (*Shi Gao*), 20g, Radix Ledebouriellae Sesloidis (*Fang Feng*), 15g, Rhizoma Coptidis Chinensis (*Huang Lian*), 10g, Herba Menthae (*Bo He*), 10g, Radix Rubrus Paeoniae Lactiflorae (*Chi Shao*), 10g, Flos Pruni Mume (*Lu O Mei*), and Radix Glycyrrhizae (*Gan Cao*), 10g. She was given 3 *ji*, decocted in water and administered.

At her second diagnosis (*i.e.*, second visit), she reported that after taking the above medicinals the swelling and pain of the lips of her mouth had very markedly diminished. However, the amount of her menses had been excessive. Therefore, 10g of Herba Artemesiae Apiaceae (*Qing Hao*) and 10g of Herba Leonuri Heterophylli (*Kun Cao*) were added to her formula and she was given 3 more *ji*. This led to her disease being cured. She used the above treatment during the week of her period for the next three months. The amount of her menstruation diminished and was without clots and her periods lasted 5 days and then stopped.

According to the author's discussion, premenstrual lip swelling and pain is not commonly seen in clinical practice. This disease is not (solely) located in the viscera and bowels, and, therefore, using (only) bitter, cold medicinals to clear heat, it is difficult to get a completely satisfactory result. This is because this disease is located within the spleen channel. The spleen opens into the portal of the mouth and its efflorescence is in the lips. In this case, there is stagnant heat in the spleen and stomach. This is due to depressive fire internally harassing. Heat tends to flame upward and this causes premenstrual swelling and pain of the lips of the mouth. After the period, this heat follows the exiting of the blood and the condition disappears. If there is heat within the body, this may also affect the two vessels, the *chong* and *ren*. This then manifests as heavy and prolonged periods. The appropriate treatment for this condition is to drain and scatter fire.

Within the formula *Xie Huang San*, raw Gypsum's acridity and coldness scatters fire, while its bitterness and coldness clear heat. In addition, it enters the spleen and stomach. Gardenia, which is bitter and cold, clears and disinhibits the three burners. Thus heat is exited via the urination. Because, in this case, heat is flaring upward in the spleen channel, Ledebouriella is used to course and scatter stagnant heat. Therefore, the upper and lower are divided and dispersed, resulting in heat being disinhibited and conducted. This is based on the principle in the *Nei Jing (Inner Classic)*, "Out-thrust depressive heat."

Agastaches fragrantly and aromatically out-thrusts and scatters. It is assisted by Ledebouriella which scatters fire. These two also arouse the spleen and harmonize the stomach. Raw Licorice drains fire and resolves toxins. It also regulates the other medicinals and harmonizes the center. Coptis is added to assist Gypsum downbear heat in the spleen/stomach. Mint and Flos Pruni Mume, which are acrid and cool, are added to scatter depressive fire. Red Peony cools the blood and regulates the menses. Artemesia Apiacea fragrantly and aromatically penetrates and scatters heat from the blood division. And Leonurus quickens the blood and transforms stasis, thus regulating the _chong_ and _ren_. Therefore, taken as a whole, this formula courses and scatters above and below. This agrees with the Ming dynasty master of medicine Wu Kun's saying:

> Use windy medicinals to scatter hidden fire. Use clearing medicinals to drain accumulations and stagnation. Combine these with sweet, relaxing (medicinals) to harmonize the center. Thus the righteous qi will not be damaged. This method is quite good.

Gynecologic _Bi Zheng_

"The Treatment of 100 Cases of Gynecologic _Bi Zheng_ with Great Supplementation of the Qi & Blood Method" by Jin Ming-mo, _Ji Lin Zhong Yi Yao (Jilin Traditional Chinese Medicine & Medicinals)_, #5, 1993, p. 27; BF

This clinical audit describes the treatment of 100 cases of gynecological _bi zheng_ using the method of greatly supplementing the qi and blood. The author treated these women between 1982-1992. This condition is called gynecological _bi zheng_ because a D&C, miscarriage, induced labor, or postpartum (condition) results in _bi zheng_. Of the 100 women, 17 had had D&C's, 9 miscarriages, 5 induced labors, 5 Caesarean births (literally, slit abdomens), and 64 normal births. Thirteen came for examination 1 week after delivery, 46 in the second week after delivery, 30 one whole month after delivery, and 11 after more than a month after delivery. Forty-five cases had generalized aching and pain in their joints. Twenty-two had low back pain. Nineteen had knee pain. And 14 had shoulder and upper arm joint pain. Ten cases had fear of wind and fear of chill. Twenty-three cases had headache and vertigo. Eight cases had shoulder, upper back, and hip pain due to wind cold external invasion. Nine cases had facial edema and 3 cases had generalized edema. Six cases had toothache, 3 cases ringing in the ears, 2 cases feet and leg pain, 3 cases eye pain, 2 cases tearing, and 3 cases spoon-shaped fingernails.

In order to greatly supplement the qi and blood, the following medicinals were used: Radix Rubrus Panacis Ginseng (*Hong Shen*), 10g, Radix Astragali Membranacei (*Huang Qi*), 100g, Semen Pruni Persicae (*Tao Ren*), 10g, Rhizoma Ligustici Wallichii (*Chuan Xiong*), 10g, Radix Angelicae Sinensis (*Dang Gui*), 10g, Radix Albus Paeoniae Lactiflorae (*Bai Shao*), 10g, Cortex Cinnamomi (*Rou Gui*), 5g, Radix Praeparatus Aconiti Carmichaeli (*Fu Zi*), 10g, Radix Angelicae Duhuo (*Du Huo*), 10g, Radix Et Rhizoma Notopterygii (*Qiang Huo*), 10g, Scolopendra Subspinipes (*Wu Gong*), 2 pieces, and Buthus Martensis (*Quan Xie*), 5g. These were decocted in water and administered 2 times per day.

If there was shoulder and upper back pain, Rhizoma Curcumae (*Jiang Huang*) was added. If there was low back pain, Radix Dipsaci (*Chuan Duan*) and Radix Achyranthis Bidentatae (*Niu Xi*) were added. If there was knee pain, Cortex Eucommiae Ulmoidis (*Du Zhong*) and Ramus Loranthi Seu Visci (*Sang Ji Sheng*) were added. If there was edema, shortness of breath, and dizziness, the amount of Astragalus was increased. If there was poor appetite, parched Three Immortals (*Jiao San Xian*) were added. If there were spoon-shaped fingernails, *Dang Gui* was added. If there were flourishing of wind evils, Zaocys Dhumnades (*Wu She*) was added, but if damp evils were victorious, Rhizoma Dioscoreae Hypoglaucae (*Bi Xie*) and Semen Coicis

Lachryma-jobi (_Yi Yi Ren_) were added. And if cold evils were flourishing, Radix Aconiti (_Chuan Wu_) was added.

Of these 100 cases, 86 were completely cured, meaning that, after treatment, their aching and pain disappeared, their movement became normal, and one half year later there was no recurrence. Ten cases received some results. This meant that their aching and pain did not completely disappear but they were able to work normally. And 4 cases experienced no results, their condition not changing from before to after treatment. Thus the total amelioration rate with this protocol was 96%.

Menstrual Pneumothorax

"A Clinical Report on the Treatment of 6 Cases of Menstrual Pneumothorax Using _Xue Fu Zhu Yu Tang_ (Dispelling Stasis from the Blood Mansion Decoction)" by Shen Guo-nan & Cheng Qun-cai, _Zhong Yi Za Zhi (Journal of Traditional Chinese Medicine)_, #11, 1993, p. 668; BF

Menstrual pneumothorax refers to either one-sided or bilateral pneumothorax occurring in women either premenstrually or during menstruation. This typically recurs each cycle. It is a rarely seen condition in clinical practice. However, since 1983, the authors have seen 6 cases of this disease which they have treated with _Xue Fu Zhu Yu Tang_ with good results.

These 6 cases were all between 14-19 years of age. They had experienced pneumothorax during their periods from 3-16 times. There were 5 cases of one-sided pneumothorax and 1 case of bilateral pneumothorax. In 4 cases, lung compression was below 30%, in 1 case 50%, and in 1 case 70%. There was no previous history of chest or lung disease. In 2 cases, examination of the pleura revealed the presence of endometriosis.

73

Xue Fu Zhu Yu Tang consists of: Semen Pruni Persicae (*Tao Ren*), 10g, Flos Carthami Tinctorii (*Hong Hua*), 10g, Radix Angelicae Sinensis (*Dang Gui*), 12g, Radix Rubrus Paeoniae Lactiflorae (*Chi Shao*), 15g, raw Radix Rehmanniae (*Sheng Di*), 12g, Rhizoma Ligustici Wallichii (*Chuan Xiong*), 15g, Radix Bupleuri (*Chai Hu*), 12g, Fructus Citri Seu Ponciri (*Zhi Ke*), 12g, Radix Platycodi Grandiflori (*Jie Geng*), 12g, Radix Achyranthis Bidentatae (*Niu Xi*), 12g, Radix Glycyrrhizae (*Gan Cao*), 10g. The above medicinals were decocted in 800ml of water, afterward reserving 600ml of liquid. One *ji* was used per day divided into 3 doses administered orally during the entire episode of pneumothorax. Afterwards, beginning 10 days before the next menstruation, 1 *ji* was administered per day through the period. If there was no recurrence of pneumothorax, these medicinals were stopped after 2 menstrual cycles.

The smallest number of *ji* administered was 7 and the largest was 15, with the average being 9 *ji*. There was no recurrence of pneumothorax after 3-5 menstrual cycles and, on follow-up after 1 year, this disease had been cured by this treatment. Thus all 6 cases were healed.

Case history: Female, student, 16 years old. This girl's menstruation had begun at 14 years of age. For the previous 6 months, 3-5 days before the onset of each period, she experienced chest oppression, rapid breathing, cough, and right-sided chest pain. She was diagnosed as suffering from right-sided pneumothorax and her lung compression was only 30% She was hospitalized for treatment for 10 days, (during which time) the gas (in her pleural cavity) was reabsorbed. Some time later her condition recurred. She experienced vexation and agitation and rapid breathing. Her lips were dark purple. Her tongue was static (colored) and dark with a thin, white coating. And her pulse was choppy/astringent and rapid. She had a stuffy feeling in the area of her right ribs and her breathing was diminished and weak. Again she was diagnosed as suffering from right-sided pneumothorax and her lung compression was 50%. Because she also experienced abdominal pain each time her period came, because her menstruation's amount was scanty and dark colored, and because her period was, to varying degrees, late, the authors diagnosed her case as suffering from menstrual pneumothorax and administered the above medicinals for 3 days, after which her period came. Its amount was scanty and color was dark. It also contained clots. Eleven *ji* later, her pneumothorax was completely reabsorbed. For the next 2 menstrual cycles, she was administered these medicinals during her period. Although she experienced a recurrence of pneumothorax, its symptoms were reduced and her lung compression was only 10% below normal. She stopped taking these medicinals after another 2 menstrual cycles and 1 year later on follow-up there had been no recurrence.

The authors say that menstrual pneumothorax may be associated with endometriosis. Because it presents with chest oppression and chest pain, rapid breathing, cough, and a suffocating feeling along with scanty menstruation which is dark colored and is accompanied by abdominal pain when the menstruation comes, it may be classified as qi stagnation, blood stasis. Therefore, its treatment should mainly consist of regulating and rectifying the qi mechanism, quickening the blood, and transforming stasis. *Xue Fu Zhu Yu Tang* is a formula which quickens the blood and transforms stasis. It treats diseases having these very disease mechanisms.

Post-menstrual Strangury

"The Treatment of Post-menstrual Strangury with *Jia Wei Lao Lin Tang* (Added Flavors Taxation Strangury Decoction)" by Ni Shi-tao, *Si Chuan Zhong Yi (Sichuan Traditional Chinese Medicine)*, #6, 1993, p. 41; BF

Since 1981, the author has treated 70 cases of post-menstrual strangury (*lin zheng*) using Zhang Jing-yue's *Lao Lin Tang* with added flavors, and, in all cases, this was completely effective. *Jia Wei Lao*

Lin Tang consists of: Radix Dioscoreae Oppositae (*Shan Yao*) and Rhizoma Imperatae Cyclindricae (*Bai Mao Gen*), 30-60g @, Herba Plantaginis (*Che Qian Cao*), 20-30g, Semen Euryalis Ferocis (*Qian Shi*) and raw Radix Astragali Membranacei (*Sheng Huang Qi*), 15-25g @, Radix Albus Paeoniae Lactiflorae (*Bai Shao*), 10-15g, Gelatinum Corii Asini (*E Jiao*), Sclerotium Polypori Umbellati (*Zhu Ling*), and Rhizoma Anemarrhenae (*Zhi Mu*), 10g @, and Radix Glycyrrhizae (*Gan Cao*), 6g.

If there was damp heat, the amount of Euryales and Astragalus was reduced and Caulis Akebiae Mutong (*Mu Tong*), Talcum (*Hua Shi*), and Cortex Phellodendri (*Huang Bai*) were added. If vacuity cold was severe, Imperata and Anemarrhena were subtracted and Ramulus Cinnamomi (*Gui Zhi*) and Rhizoma Curculiginis Orchoidis (*Xian Mao*) were added. If there was copious blood in the urine, Herba Cephalanopolos Segeti (*Xiao Ji*), raw Radix Rehmanniae (*Sheng Di*), and carbonized Pollen Typhae (*Pu Huang Tan*) were added. If there was lower abdominal distention and fullness, Radix Saussureae Seu Vladimiriae (*Mu Xiang*) and Rhizoma Cyperi Rotundi (*Xiang Fu*) were added. If there was low back and knee soreness and weakness, Radix Achyranthis Bidentatae (*Huai Niu Xi*), prepared Radix Rehmanniae (*Shu Di*), and Cortex Eucommiae Ulmoidis (*Du Zhong*) were added. These were decocted in water and administered, 1 *ji* per day. Administration began 5 days before the period and continued to the period. Approximately 10-14 *ji* equalled 1 course of treatment.

Case history: Chen, female, 36 years old. Each month after her period, this woman would experience urinary frequency and urgency accompanied by a burning hot, unsmooth feeling. For the previous 3 years, after each menstruation she had used antibiotics and vitamins B_1 and B_6 which reduced the symptoms somewhat. Currently, before each period, she felt spiritual exhaustion and bodily fatigue. In addition, she had a dry throat and heart vexation, a pale tongue with thin, yellow coating, and a fine, rapid pulse. This pattern was categorized as spleen/kidney dual vacuity with vacuity heat harassing internally and the qi transformation not disinhibited. The treatment principles were to fortify the spleen and boost the kidneys, enrich yin and clear heat, and open strangury.

The formula used was _Jia Wei Lao Lin Tang_: Radix Dioscoreae Oppositae (_Shan Yao_) and Rhizoma Imperatae Cylindricae (_Bai Mao Gen_), 30g @, raw Radix Astragali Membranacei (_Sheng Huang Qi_), 20g, Semen Euryalis Ferocis (_Qian Shi_) and Herba Plantaginis (_Che Qian Cao_), 25g @, Radix Albus Paeoniae Lactiflorae (_Bai Shao_), Gelatinum Corii Asini (_E Jiao_), Rhizoma Anemarrhenae (_Zhi Mu_), and Sclerotium Polypori Umbellati (_Zhu Ling_), 10g @, and Radix Glycyrrhizae (_Gan Cao_), 6g. The patient was given 3 _ji_ and then the period came and the medicinals were stopped. Three day after the period stopped, 3 _ji_ of the previous formula were given and the symptoms disappeared. However, there was still low back and knee soreness and weakness. Therefore, 15g of Cortex Eucommiae Ulmoidis (_Du Zhong_) and 25g @ of Radix Achyranthis Bidentatae (_Huai Niu Xi_) and prepared Radix Rehmanniae (_Shu Di_) were added to the above formula. She was given 8 _ji_, 5 of which she took then and 3 of which she took before her next period. After 1 course of treatment, she was cured and there was no recurrence after 2 years.

According to Dr. Ni's discussion, this condition corresponds to a urinary tract infection in Western medicine. In TCM, after the period, the qi and blood are both deficient. During this period, the liver and kidneys may lose their regulation and the bladder qi may lose its control with heat being retained within the bladder. The _Zhu Bing Yuan Hou Lun (Treatise on the Cause & Symptoms of Disease)_ states,

> Strangury is caused by kidney vacuity and heat in the bladder...Kidney vacuity leads to the urination being numerous. Heat in the bladder leads to water's descent being astringent. This then leads to dribbling which is not diffused and this is what is called strangury.

Therefore, this formula with its added ingredients supplements the kidneys and fortifies the spleen, boosts the qi and enriches yin, and clears heat and opens strangury. It supports the righteous without retaining evils and it disperses evils without damaging the righteous.

Perimenstrual Hemoptysis

"One Case of Menstrual Movement Coughing Up Blood" by Zhang Xin, *Ji Lin Zhong Yi Yao (Jilin Chinese Medicine & Medicinals)*, #4, 1993, p. 28; BF

The patient was an 18 year old female student. For the past 4 months she had been coughing up blood with her period. (This is a symptom of endometriosis.) Menarche had occurred at 15 years of age and her periods had been normal until the last half year when she had been studying too hard and overworking her brain. This had resulted in excessive thinking, worry, and anxiety accompanied by dizziness, heart vexation, loss of sleep, and excessive dreaming. She administered herself *Jian Nao Bu Xin Wan* (Fortify the Brain, Supplement the Heart Pills), *Shen Qi Da Bu Wan* (Ginseng & Astragalus Great Supplement Pills), and other such medicines but without result.

Four months earlier, during her period, she suddenly felt that her throat was not right and subsequently coughed up and spit out 5ml of blood from her mouth. Mixed in with this were a small amount of phlegm fluids. After coughing up this blood, the feeling of something not right in her throat disappeared and there was no cough, vomiting, fever, or other such symptoms. Her menses was red in color and its amount was normal. However, it was accompanied by a light degree of lower abdominal distention and pain. After this, each day she coughed up 3-5ml of blood, 2-4 times per day without other symptoms. After the period was over, the coughing up blood stopped.

The young woman underwent various Western medical examinations and was given vitamin K₄ and *San Qi Fen* (Pseudoginseng Powder). After several months, she came for a TCM diagnosis. This revealed that her essence spirit was repressed and her depression was not aroused. Her tongue was red with a thin, yellow coating. Her pulse was wiry, thready, and rapid. These symptoms are categorized as liver depression and internal heat, yin vacuity and yang hyperactivity. Therefore, treatment should course the liver and resolve depression, nourish yin and clear heat, as well as lead the blood downward in movement.

Thus, *Qing Jing Si Wu Tang* combined with *Dan Zhi Xiao Yao San* with additions and subtractions was used: Radix Rehmanniae (*Sheng Di*), Radix Albus Paeoniae Lactiflorae (*Bai Shao*), Herba Ecliptae Prostratae (*Han Lian Cao*), and Haematitum (*Dai Zhe Shi*), 20g each, Radix Angelicae Sinensis (*Dang Gui*), Rhizoma Anemarrhenae (*Zhi Mu*), and Radix Cyathulae (*Chuan Niu Xi*), 12g each, Cortex Radicis Moutan (*Mu Dan Pi*), Fructus Gardeniae Jasminoidis (*Zhi Zi*), Fructus Arctii (*Niu Bang Zi*), Rhizoma Cyperi Rotundi (*Xiang Fu*), and Radix Polygalae Tenuifoliae (*Yuan Zhi*), 10g each, Radix Bupleuri (*Chai Hu*), 8g, and Rhizoma Imperatae Cylindricae (*Bai Mao Gen*), 30g. These were decocted in water and taken. Each day 1 *ji* was taken in 2 divided doses.

After taking 3 *ji* of the above prescription, the menstrual period ceased and the coughing up blood also stopped automatically. Then the patient was given *Tian Wang Bu Xin Wan* (Heavenly King Supplement the Heart Pills) combined with *Xiao Yao Wan* (Rambling Pills). Three days before the onset of the next period, she was again given the above formula for the following 7 days. During the 5 days of her period, she coughed up blood 3 times. Its amount was scanty and less than before. She also experienced dizziness, heart vexation, and loss of sleep. She was advised how to pay attention to essence spirit regulation and discipline. She was administered 2 courses of the above method of treatment. One half year later on follow-up, the patient reported that she had had no recurrence of coughing up blood.

Amenorrhea

"65 Cases of Amenorrhea Treated with *Gua Shi Liu Wei Tang* (Trichosanthes & Dendrobium Six Flavors Decoction" by Tang Kun-hua & Zhu Guang-hua, *Jiang Su Zhong Yi (Jiangsu Traditional Chinese Medicine)*, #11, 1993, p. 9; BF

This clinical audit reports on the treatment of 65 cases of amenorrhea using *Gua Shi Liu Wei Tang* over several years. The ages of the patients ranged from 16-47 years with an average age of 30.5 years of age. Among these women, the shortest duration of amenorrhea was 3 months and the longest was 10 years. In terms of their *bian zheng* diagnosis, 26 cases were categorized as yin vacuity with blood heat, 17 cases as qi stagnation and blood stasis, 10 cases as imbalance of the liver and spleen, 7 cases as liver/kidney insufficiency, and 5 cases as phlegm dampness obstruction and stagnation. In this audit, all the women experienced a resumption of normal menstruation within 3 months of treatment and were thus considered cured.

Gua Shi Liu Wei Tang is composed of: Fructus Trichosanthis Kirlowii (*Quan Gua Lou*), Herba Dendrobii (*Shi Hu*), Herba Leonuri Heterophylli (*Yi Mu Cao*), Cortex Radicis Moutan (*Dan Pi*), Radix Salviae Miltiorrhizae (*Dan Shen*), and Radix Achyranthis Bidentatae (*Niu Xi*). Each day, 1 prescription decocted in water and divided into 2 doses.

If the patient's pattern was yin vacuity with blood heat, Radix Rehmanniae (*Sheng Di*), Radix Scrophulariae Ningpoensis (*Xuan Shen*), Tuber Ophiopogonis Japonicae (*Mai Dong*), and Rhizoma Coptidis Chinensis (*Huang Lian*) were added. If the patient's pattern was qi stagnation and blood stasis, Radix Bupleuri (*Chai Hu*), Fructus Citri Seu Ponciri (*Zhi Qiao*), Rhizoma Cyperi Rotundi (*Xiang Fu*), Semen Biotae Orientalis (*Bai Zi Ren*), Herba Lycopi Lucidi (*Ze Lan*), Semen Vaccariae Segetalis (*Wang Bu Liu Xing*), and Herba Selaginellae Tamariscinae (*Juan Bo*) were added. If the patient's pattern was imbalance of the liver and spleen, Radix Bupleuri (*Chai Hu*), Rhizoma Atractylodis Macrocephalae (*Bai Zhu*), Radix Ledebouriellae Sesloidis (*Fang Feng*), Rhizoma Cyperi Rotundi (*Xiang Fu*), Sclerotium Poriae Cocos (*Fu Ling*), Pericarpium Viridis Citri Reticulatae (*Qing Pi*), and Pericarpium Citri Reticulatae (*Chen Pi*) were added. If the patient's pattern was liver/kidney insufficiency, Radix Rehmanniae (*Sheng Di*), prepared Radix Rehmanniae (*Shu Di*), Radix Dioscoreae Oppositae (*Shan Yao*), Fructus Corni Officinalis (*Zhu Rou*), Radix Dipsaci (*Chuan Duan*), and Radix Morindae (*Ba Ji*) were added. And if the patient's pattern was phlegm dampness obstruction and stagnation, Rhizoma Pinelliae Ternatae (*Fa Ban Xia*), Sclerotium Poriae Cocos (*Fu Ling*), aged bile(-processed) Rhizoma Arisaematis (*Chen Dan Xing*), Rhizoma Atractylodis (*Cang Zhu*), and Caulis In Taeniis Bambusae (*Zhu Ru*) were added.

According to Tang and Zhu, this formula enriches yin and clears heat, loosens the chest and transforms phlegm, moistens dryness and harmonizes the stomach, and quickens the blood and frees the channels. In particular, Trichosanthes loosens the chest and scatters nodulation, transforms phlegm and moistens dryness. Dendrobium enriches yin and nourishes the stomach, generates fluids and eliminates heat. Leonurus quickens the blood and dispels stasis, generates fluids and regulates the menses. Moutan clears heat and cools the blood, quickens the blood and scatters stasis. Salvia quickens the blood and transforms stasis, cools the blood and regulates the menses. And Achyranthis quickens the blood and expels stasis, supplements the kidneys and frees the channels. As a whole, this formula is for the treatment of yin vacuity with stomach heat. In this case, scorching heat has injured stomach fluids and humors. Thus the *chong* and *ren* lose their balance and menses is emitted only rarely. After some time, the essence and blood become consumed and exhausted and, therefore, there is amenorrhea.

Meno-metrorrhagia

"A Comparative Study of the Treatment of Spleen/Kidney Yang Vacuity Pattern Functional Uterine Bleeding (Using) Warming the Kidneys & Strengthening the Spleen Methods" by Fu You-feng *et al.*, *Jiang Su Zhong Yi (Jiangsu Traditional Chinese Medicine)*, #11, 1993, p. 7-8; BF

The authors begin this study saying that functional uterine bleeding corresponds to what is called flooding and leakage, early menstruation, or menstruation before, after or at no fixed interval in TCM. They then go on to compare the TCM treatment of 53 cases of specifically spleen/kidney yang vacuity functional bleeding to a control group of 19 patients treated with modern Western medicine. Among the group treated with Chinese medicine, 9 were adolescents, 26 were of child-bearing age, and 18 were menopausal. Among the control group, 4 were adolescents, 9 were of child-bearing age, and 6 were menopausal.

The criteria for these patient's TCM pattern discrimination diagnosis included excessive bleeding from the vaginal tract or dribbling and dripping of blood without cease. The color of the blood was pale red, and its consistency was dilute and without clots. Patient's faces were ashen white, and their bodies were cold and limbs chilled. In addition, they suffered from low back and knee soreness and weakness or low back pain as if about to break, not enough warmth in their four limbs or edematous swelling, long, clear urination, and loose stools. Their tongues were pale red and swollen with the indentations of their teeth along their edges. The coating was thin and white. Their pulses were deep, fine, without force, etc.

The Chinese herbal treatment was based on the principles of warming the kidneys and fortifying the spleen, boosting the qi and stopping bleeding. The formula consisted of: Fructus Psoraleae Corylifoliae (*Bu

Gu Zhi), Os Sepiae Seu Sepiellae (*Wu Zei Gu*), Cortex Cinnamomi (*Rou Gui*), Radix Angelicae Sinensis (*Dang Gui*), processed Rhizoma Cyperi Rotundi (*Zhi Xiang Fu*), Radix Codonopsis Pilosulae (*Dang Shen*), Radix Astragali Membranacei (*Huang Qi*), and raw Rhizoma Atractylodis Macrocephalae (*Sheng Bai Zhu*). Each day, one *ji* or formula was given unless the case was serious, in which case 2 *ji* were given. These herbs were given during the time of the bleeding and then again for 3 days before the next period arrived. The control group received *Zi Xue An* (Uterine Bleeding Quieter, active ingredients unspecified), 4 pills 3 times per day. Typically bleeding stopped after 4-7 days of herbs with the longest requiring 10 days. The course of treatment lasted 3 whole months.

The definition of results were as follows: Marked results consisted of return of the amount of menstrual blood to normal or diminishment by more than half and bleeding stopping within 7 days. Good results consisted of the amount of menstrual blood being reduced to from 1/3-1/2 and bleeding stopping in from 8-10 days. No results meant that the amount of menstrual blood was not diminished. Based on these definitions, among those treated with Chinese herbs and whose bleeding was reduced in volume, 36 cases experienced marked results, 15 experienced good results, and 2 cases experienced no results. This gives a total amelioration rate *vis á vis* reduction of the amount of bleeding of 96.2%. This compares with a total amelioration rate *vis á vis* reduction of blood volume in the comparison group of only 78.9%. In terms of shortening the length of the period, 47 women in the Chinese herb group experienced marked results, 4 experienced good results, and 2 experienced no results for the same amelioration rate of 96.2% as compared to a total amelioration rate in the comparison group of only 36.8%.

"The Treatment of 124 Cases of Pubescent 'Stirring Blood' by the Methods of Boosting the Qi, Nourishing Yin, and Securing the Menses" by Zou Qi, *Shang Hai Zhong Yi Yao Za Zhi (The Shanghai Journal of Traditional Chinese Medicine & Medicinals)*, # 6, 1993, p. 16-17; BF

The author begins this clinical audit by saying that pubescent functional uterine bleeding is a commonly seen disease in gynecology departments. In Traditional Chinese Medicine, it is categorized as *beng lou* or flooding and leaking. If the bleeding is excessive in quantity and pours downward, this is *beng* or flooding, while if it is scanty in amount and continuously dribbles, this is *lou* or leakage. Since 1988, the author has treated 124 cases of this condition using the methods of boosting the qi, nourishing yin, and securing the menses. All these patients were between 13-18 years old, with 12 cases being 13, 28 cases 14, 34 cases 15, 27 cases 16, 14 cases 17, and 9 cases being 18 years of age. The onset of this disease had occurred from 6 months to 4 years after menarche, with the average being 1-2 years after menarche. In most of these patients, their menstrual cycle was 15-23 days. In 56 cases, their period was 7-10 days long and in 28 cases, it was 11-15 days long. In 6 which were severe, flooding and leaking were continuous. Other symptoms included dizziness, spiritual fatigue, lack of strength, diminished facial lustre or a faded yellow complexion, reduced appetite, possible abdominal pain, a pale tongue with red tongue tip, and a fine, rapid pulse.

Treatment was divided into two phases. During the intermenstruum, the treatment principles were to boost the qi and nourish yin using: Radix Astragali Membranacei (*Huang Qi*), 30g, Radix Codonopsis Pilosulae (*Dang Shen*), Rhizoma Atractylodis Macrocephalae (*Bai Zhu*), raw Radix Rehmanniae (*Sheng Di*), Radix Albus Paeoniae Lactiflorae (*Bai Shao*), Fructus Ligustri Lucidi (*Nu Zhen Zi*), Herba Ecliptae Prostratae (*Han Lian Cao*), and Rhizoma Anemarrhenae (*Zhi Mu*), 10g @. At the same time, patients were also required to take *Wu Ji Bai Feng Wan* (Black Chicken, White Phoenix Pills).

During the period itself, depending upon the amount of menses and the duration of the period, the above formula with various additions and subtractions was given. Commonly, raw Pollen Typhae (*Sheng Pu Huang*), 10-20g, carbonized Radix Sanguisorbae (*Di Yu Tan*), 30g, Cortex Cedrelae (*Chun Gen Bai Pi*), Os Sepiae Seu Sepiellae (*Wu Zei Gu*), and Radix Rubiae Cordifoliae (*Qian Cao*), 10-15g, were added in order to secure the menses. Administration of these medicinals for 3 whole months equalled 1 course of treatment.

Complete cure consisted of the amount of menstruation and its cycle returning to normal with no recurrence in 3 whole menstrual cycles after stopping the medicinals. Improvement consisted of the amount and duration of the period returning to normal but not being able to maintain this normalcy for 3 whole months after stopping these medicinals or shortening of the period and reduction of the amount of blood. No result was defined as no apparent change in the patient's condition after 3 months of treatment. Based on these criteria, 84 young women were cured, 31 got some improvement, and 9 experienced no result.

According to the author, this condition is primarily due to *chong* and *ren* vacuity detriment and lack of security of the *chong* and *ren*. The *chong* is the sea of blood and the *ren* controls the *bao tai* (uterus & fetus). If these two vessels suffer vacuity detriment, they will not be able to hold the blood within the channels and thus there is *beng lou* below. In the case of pubescent stirring of blood, kidney water is deficient and water deficiency leads to fire effulgence. Heat is hidden in the *chong* and *ren* and this heat harasses and stirs the *bao mai*.

Premenstrual Breast Distention, Fibrocystic Breast Disease, & Benign Breast Lumps

"The Pattern Discrimination Treatment of 90 Cases of Menstrual Movement Breast Distention" by Wang Fa-chang & Wang Qu-an, *Shan Dong Zhong Yi Za Zhi (The Shandong Journal of Traditional Chinese Medicine)*, **#5, 1993, p. 24-5; BF**

Menstrual movement, *i.e.*, perimenstrual, breast distention and pain is one of the most commonly seen complaints in gynecology departments. The authors of this clinical audit have treated 90 cases of this condition based on pattern discrimination. Of these 90 women, 4 were between 16-20 years old, 11 between 21-25, 20 between 26-30, 21 between 31-35, 20 between 36-40, 5 between 41-45, 7 between 46-50, and 2 cases were more than 50 years old. The course of these women's disease was from one half year to 20 years.

1. Simultaneous liver depression with damp heat pattern

The main symptoms of this pattern were premenstrual chest oppression, heart vexation and easy anger, breast distention and pain, a dry mouth, vexatious heat of the chest and epigastrium, lower abdominal aching and pain, possible vaginal itching or excessive, yellow-colored vaginal discharge, a wiry, rapid pulse, and red tongue with a thin, yellow coating. The treatment principles were to course the liver and resolve depression, clear heat and disinhibit dampness. The formula consisted of a combination of *Dan Zhi Xiao Yao San* (Moutan & Gardenia Rambling Powder), *Yi Huang Tang* (Change Yellow [Discharge] Decoction), and *San Miao San* (Three Wonders Powder) plus Rhizoma Cyperi Rotundi (*Xiang Fu*).

2. Simultaneous liver depression with blood stasis pattern

The main symptoms of this pattern were premenstrual heart vexation and easy anger, breast distention and pain, occasional nodulation, lower abdominal distention and pain disliking pressure, possible scanty menstruation which does not come smoothly, a dark, purplish menstruate containing clots, a wiry, slippery pulse, and a purplish, dark tongue with static spots or patches and a thin, white coating. The treatment principles were to course the liver and resolve depression, quicken the blood, transform stasis, and stop pain. The formula consisted of *Dan Zhi Xiao Yao San* (Moutan & Gardenia Rambling Powder) combined with *Tao Hong Si Wu Tang* (Persica & Carthamus Four Materials Decoction) plus Pericarpium Viridis Citri Reticulatae (*Qing Pi*), Rhizoma Corydalis Yanhusuo (*Yan Hu Suo*), and Tuber Curcumae (*Yu Jin*).

3. Simultaneous liver depression with heart/spleen dual vacuity pattern

The main symptoms of this pattern were premenstrual chest oppression, heart vexation and chaotic thoughts, mild, insidious breast pain or small sensations of distention, heart palpitations, dizziness, loss of sleep, excessive dreams, lack of strength of the entire body, spiritual exhaustion, diminished appetite, excessive, pasty white vaginal discharge, a wiry, fine pulse, and a pale tongue with teethmarks on its border and a thin, white coating. The treatment principles were to course the liver and resolve depression, fortify the spleen and harmonize the stomach, nourish the heart and quiet the spirit. The formula consisted of *Dan Shen Gui Pi Tang* (Salvia Restore the Spleen Decoction) plus Rhizoma Cyperi Rotundi (*Xiang Fu*) and Tuber Curcumae (*Yu Jin*).

4. Liver/kidney insufficiency pattern

The main symptoms of this pattern were premenstrual chest oppression, heart vexation and chaotic thoughts, mild, insidious breast pain, dizziness, tinnitus, low back pain, weakness of the extremities, lack of strength, a deep, wiry pulse, and a pale tongue with scant coating. The treatment principles were to course the liver and fortify the spleen, supplement and boost the liver and kidneys. The formula consisted of *Dan Zhi Xiao Yao San* (Moutan & Gardenia Rambling Powder) plus Cortex Eucommiae Ulmoidis (*Du Zhong*), Radix Dipsaci (*Chuan Xu Duan*), Ramus Loranthi Seu Visci (*Sang Ji Sheng*), Cornu Degelatinum Cervi (*Lu Jiao Shuang*), Fructus Corni Officinalis (*Shan Zhu Yu*), and Semen Cuscutae (*Tu Si Zi*).

5. Simultaneous liver depression with *chong* and *ren* vacuity cold pattern

The main symptoms of this pattern were premenstrual heart vexation and chaotic thoughts, spiritual exhaustion, breast distention and pain, insidious lower abdominal pain with a cool sensation, a fine, slow pulse, and a pale tongue with a thin, white coating. The treatment principles were to course the liver and resolve depression, cherish the palace (*i.e.*, uterus) and scatter cold. The formula consisted of *Dan Zhi Xiao Yao San* (Moutan & Gardenia Rambling Powder) plus Radix Linderae Strychnifoliae (*Wu Yao*), Rhizoma Cyperi Rotundi (*Xiang Fu*), stir-fried Fructus Foeniculi Vulgaris (*Chao Xiao Hui*), and stir-fried Folium Artemesiae Argyii (*Chao Ai Ye*).

One course of treatment was comprised of 3 *ji* of the appropriate Chinese medicinals being given during the premenstruum. Complete cure was defined as disappearance of such symptoms as premenstrual chest oppression, heart vexation and chaotic thoughts, breast distention and pain, etc. with reduction or disappearance of nodulations and lumps in the breasts within 3 courses of treatment. Marked improvement consisted of reduction in such symptoms as premenstrual chest oppression, heart vexation and chaotic thoughts, breast distention and pain, etc. within 3 courses of treatment. Good improvement consisted of reduction in the same sorts of symptoms as above in 3 courses of treatment but recurrence or worsening of these symptoms due emotional stress. Of the 90 women treated in this study, 57 were cured, 23 were marked improved, 8 experienced good improvement, and 2 got no result. Thus the total amelioration rate using this protocol was 97.8%.

"The Treatment of 24 Cases of Mammary Hyperplasia with *Ru Kuai Xiao Tang Jia Wei* (Breast Lump Dispersing Decoction with Added Flavors" by Hou Jian, *Shan Dong Zhong Yi Za Zhi (The Shandong Journal of Traditional Chinese Medicine)*, #5, 1993, p. 33; BF

This clinical audit reports on the treatment of 24 cases of mammary hyperplasia with *Ru Kuai Xiao Tang Jia Wei* from 1989-1991. The age of the women in this study ranged from 23-50 years old, with 6 cases being between 23-30, 15 between 31-40, and 3 between 41-50 years of age. Thirteen cases had suffered from this condition for within 6 months, 5 cases from 7 months to 1 year, and 6 cases for over 1 year. All these women were married. Treatment used a basic formula which was modified based on pattern discrimination.

1. Liver qi depression & stagnation pattern (13 cases)

The signs and symptoms of this pattern included breast distention and pain which occurred either before the period or got worse with the approach of the period, pain and distention reaching the chest and lateral costal regions, palpable mammary hyperplasia and lumps but without clearly demarcated borders, lumps may be changeable, lack of ease in emotional affairs, sighing, chest oppression, a darkish pale tongue with a thin, white coating, and a wiry, fine pulse.

2. Phlegm congelation, blood stasis pattern (7 cases)

The signs and symptoms of this pattern included dull breast pain and numbness. However, in prolonged cases, there was piercing pain. In addition there were nodular lumps but not adhering to the underside of the skin, pliable and not hard, typically physical fatigue, nausea, vomiting of phlegmy saliva, a gloomy (*i.e.*, darkish) tongue with a glossy, slimy coating, and a slippery or choppy/astringent pulse.

3. *Chong* & *ren* loss of regulation pattern (4 cases)

The signs and symptoms of this pattern included breast heaviness and pain, many breast lumps spread all over the place occurring with menstruation, after, or before, emotional tenseness, agitation, and easy anger, low back soreness, lack of strength, a pale tongue with a white coating, and a soggy or vacuous pulse. This pattern mostly occurred in older women.

Ru Kuai Xiao Tang consists of: Fructus Trichosanthis Kirlowii (*Gua Lou*), 15g, raw Concha Ostreae (*Sheng Mu Li*), 15g, Spica Prunellae Vulgaris (*Xia Gu Cao*), 15g, Thallus Algae (*Kun Bu*), 15g, Herba Sargassii (*Hai Zao*), Radix Salviae Miltiorrhizae (*Dan Shen*), 15g, Radix Bupleuri (*Chai Hu*), 9g, Tuber Asparagi Cochinensis (*Tian Men Dong*), 9g, Rhizoma Sparganii (*San Leng*), 9g, Rhizoma Curcumae Zedoariae (*E Zhu*), 9g, Folium Citri (*Ju Ye*), 9g, Semen Citri (*Ju He*), 9g, and Rhizoma Pinelliae Ternatae (*Ban Xia*), 9g. These were decocted in water and administered in two divided doses, 1 *ji* per day. Treatment was commenced 15 days before the onset of the period, with 12 days equalling 1 course of treatment. Administration of these medicinals was discontinued during the period.

If the pattern was liver qi depression & stagnation, Pericarpium Viridis Citri Reticulatae (*Qing Pi*) and Rhizoma Cyperi Rotundi (*Xiang Fu*), 9g @, were added to move the qi and scatter depression. If the pattern was phlegm congelation & blood stasis, the amounts of Oyster Shell, Algae, and Salvia were increased up to 30g @ to soften the hard and dispel stasis. If the pattern was *chong* & *ren* loss of regulation, Radix Morindae (*Ba Ji Tian*), Cornu Degelatinum Cervi (*Lu Jiao Shuang*), and Retinervus Luffae Cyclindricae (*Si Gua Luo*) were added to secure the kidneys, rectify the *chong*, and open the connecting vessels.

Complete cure consisted of disappearance of the breast lumps, complete reduction in the aching and pain, and no recurrence on follow-up a half year later. Some improvement was defined as reduction in the size of the lumps and diminishment in the aching and pain. No results meant that there was no change in either the lumps of the pain. Based on these criteria, in 1 course of treatment, 6 women were cured and 4 got some improvement. In 2 courses of treatment, 3 women were cured and 2 got some improvement. In 3 courses of treatment, 3 women were cured and 1 got some improvement. And in 4 courses of treatment, 1 was cured, 2 improved, and 2 got no result. Therefore, the total number of cases cured was 13. The total number of cases improved was 9. And only 2 women experienced no result. Thus the total amelioration rate was 91.7%.

Dr. Hou says that the incidence of this condition is relatively high in younger women. It is also called breast *pi*. The *Wai Ke Zheng Zong (The True Lineage of External Medicine)* states:

> Breast *pi* consists of nodulations within the breast, their form being like that of an egg. They may be heavy and painful or there may be no pain. The skin (above them) is not changed. These kernels' growth and decline may follow the (growth and decline of) joy and anger. They are mostly due to worry and anxiety damaging the spleen and irritation and anger damaging the liver with depression binding becoming (nodulation).

The author goes on to say that this protocol mainly courses the liver and resolves depression, transforms phlegm and scatters nodulation. At the same time, it also rectifies the *chong* and *ren*. Within this formula, Bupleurum, Green Orange Peel, and Orange Leaves course the liver and resolve depression. Oyster Shell, Algae, Prunella, Orange Seed, Trichosanthes, and Pinellia transform phlegm, soften the hard, and scatter nodulation. Salvia, Sparganum, and Zedoaria quicken the blood and dispel stasis. While Asparagus clears heat and dispels phlegm which is the priority treatment for this disease. When qi is moved, phlegm is dispelled, and, when blood is quickened, stasis is dispersed. Thus the disease is cured. In a small number of cases with this condition, prolonged emotional disturbance may result in liver vacuity and dry blood. In that case, the nodulations will be especially hard and the hyperplasia will be lumpy. In such cases, internal medication alone may not be adequate. Therefore, such patients should be treated with a combination of surgery, external and internal treatment, and support of the righteous while dispelling evils. Then the formula will be able to achieve results.

"50 Cases Treated for Premenstrual Breast Distention & Pain with Jie Yu Huo Xue Tang (Resolve Depression & Activate the Blood Decoction)" by Gu Si-yun, Shan Dong Zhong Yi Za Zhi (The Shandong Journal of Traditional Chinese Medicine), # 6, 1992, p. 27-8; BF

The author of this study posits that premenstrual breast distention is primarily due to liver depression and qi stagnation with subsequent loss of harmony and descension of the stomach. Since the breasts are primarily circulated by the liver and stomach channels, qi depression and stagnation affecting these two organs make it difficult for the qi to drain from these channels as they should. Fifty women suffering from premenstrual breast distention and pain were, therefore, treated with the following formula: Radix Bupleuri (Chai Hu), 12g, Rhizoma Cyperi Rotundi (Xiang Fu), 15g, Rhizoma Ligustici Wallichii (Chuan Xiong), 12g, Fructus Citri Seu Ponciri (Zhi Ke), 9g, Radix Rubrus Paeoniae Lactiflorae (Chi Shao), 12g, Semen Pruni Persicae (Tao Ren), 10g, Flos Carthami Tinctorii (Hong Hua), 9g, Pericarpium Viridis

Citri Reticulatae (*Qing Pi*), 10g, Folium Citri (*Ju Ye*), Fructus Trichosanthis Kirlowii (*Gua Lou*), 15g, Radix Glycyrrhizae (*Gan Cao*), 6g, Radix Salviae Miltiorrhizae (*Dan Shen*), 15g, Tuber Curcumae (*Yu Jin*), 12g, Radix Dioscoreae Oppositae (*Shan Yao*), 12g.

If patients suffered from spleen vacuity, Radix Codonopsis Pilosulae (*Dang Shen*), Radix Astragali Membranacei (*Huang Qi*), Rhizoma Atractylodis (*Cang Zhu*), Rhizoma Atractylodis Macrocephalae (*Bai Zhu*), and Fructus Amomi (*Sha Ren*) were added. If patients suffered from blood vacuity, Radix Angelicae Sinensis (*Dang Gui*), prepared Radix Rehmanniae (*Shu Di*), and Radix Albus Paeoniae Lactiflorae (*Bai Shao*) were added. If patients suffered from kidney yang vacuity, Cortex Eucommiae Ulmoidis (*Du Zhong*), Semen Cuscutae (*Tu Si Zi*), Radix Dipsaci (*Xu Duan*), and Herba Epimedii (*Yin Yang Huo*) were added. If patients suffered from kidney yin vacuity, Rhizoma Anemarrhenae (*Zhi Mu*), Radix Rehmanniae (*Sheng Di*), Fructus Corni Officinalis (*Shan Zhu Yu*), and Herba Ecliptae Prostratae (*Han Lian Cao*) were added. For liver fire invading the stomach, Fructus Gardeniae Jasminoidis (*Zhi Zi*), Cortex Radicis Moutan (*Dan Pi*), and Pericarpium Citri Reticulatae (*Chen Pi*) were added. For liver yang hyperactivity above, Ramulus Uncariae Cum Uncis (*Gou Teng*), Concha Margaritiferae (*Zhen Zhu Mu*), Radix Gentianae Scabrae (*Long Dan Cao*), and Flos Chrysanthemi Morifolii (*Ju Hua*) were added. For yin vacuity and yang hyperactivity, Concha Ostreae (*Mu Li*), Gelatinum Corii Asini (*E Jiao*), Tuber Ophiopogonis Japonicae (*Mai Dong*), and Radix Rehmanniae (*Sheng Di*) were added. If there was blood stasis and phlegm congelation, Radix Angelicae Sinensis (*Dang Gui*), Squama Manitis (*Chuan Shan Jia*), Semen Vaccariae Segetalis (*Wang Bu Liu Xing*), and Rhizoma Sparganii (*San Leng*) were added. These ingredients were decocted in water and one *ji* or formula, *i.e.*, packet of the above herbal medicinals, were given per day.

Of the women treated in this study, the oldest was 35 and the youngest was 15 years of age. Twenty women were between the ages of 15 and

20. Eighteen were between the ages of 21 and 30, and 12 were 31 or older. The duration of their disease had lasted from a minimum of 6 months to a maximum of 10 years with the average being 3 years. The above treatment was given for 3 whole months. At the end of that time, 44 cases or 88% experienced complete cure. Another 5 cases or 10% experienced some improvement. While only a single case or 2% failed to experience any improvement. Thus the total amelioration rate of the patients participating in this study was 98%.

"The Treatment of 128 Cases of Mammary Hyperplasia" by Mi Yang, *Hu Nan Zhong Yi Za Zhi (The Hunan Journal of Traditional Chinese Medicine)*, #1, 1993, p. 47; BF

This clinical audit describes the treatment of 128 cases of mammary hyperplasia (*i.e.*, fibrocystic breast disease) using a formula called *Shen Xiao Gua Lou San*. Traditionally, this condition was referred to as *ru pi*, breast elusive mass. Sixty-eight cases involved women between the ages of 22-30, 46 cases, 31-40, and 14 cases, 41-55 years of age.

The formula used was *Shen Xiao Gua Lou San* (Magically Dispersing Trichosanthes Powder): Fructus Trichosanthis Kirlowii (*Quan Gua Lou*), 15g, processed Gummum Olibani (*Zhi Ru Xiang*) and processed Myrrha (*Zhi Mo Yao*), 10g @, Radix Angelicae Sinensis (*Dang Gui*), 12g, and Radix Glycyrrhizae (*Gan Cao*), 6g. These were decocted in 500 ml of water, 1 *ji* or packet per day, taken in 2 divided doses.

If it was possible to feel swelling and lumps within the breast and the emotions were not easy and if there were chest and lateral costal bitterness (*i.e.*, pain) and fullness, heart vexation and easy anger, premenstrual breast distention and pain, swelling and lumps which felt achy and painful as if heavy, and pressure caused serious pain, then Radix Bupleuri (*Chai Hu*), Radix Rubrus Paeoniae Lactiflorae (*Chi Shao*), Semen Vaccariae Segetalis (*Wang Bu Liu Xing*), and stir-fried Fructus Citri Seu Ponciri (*Chao Zhi Qiao*) were added to this formula.

If the breast lumps were stringy or ropy within the breasts or scattered throughout the breasts, if their nature was pliable but tough, menstruation was excessive but pale in color, the four limbs were without strength, and there were dizziness and vertigo, Radix Astragali Membranacei (*Huang Qi*), Radix Codonopsis Pilosulae (*Dang Shen*), and Fructus Liquidambaris Taiwaniae (*Lu Lu Tong*) were added. If the breasts were swollen and painful and scorching hot, the tongue was red with a thin, yellow coating, and the pulse was wiry and rapid, Flos Lonicerae Japonicae (*Jin Yin Hua*), Fructus Forsythiae Suspensae (*Lian Qiao*), and Herba Cum Radice Taraxaci Mongolici (*Pu Gong Ying*) were added. If the breast lumps were comparatively firm but not hard, if pressure caused aching and pain, and the lumps shifted position when pushed, blast-fried Squama Manitis Pentadactylis (*Pao Shan Jia*), Spina Gleditschiae Chinensis (*Jiao Ci*), Rhizoma Sparganii (*San Leng*), and Rhizoma Curcumae Zedoariae (*E Zhu*) were added.

Treatment lasted between 30-180 days with the average being 50 days. Complete cure was defined as disappearance of the lumps. Marked improvement was defined as diminishment of the pain and aching and decrease in size of the lumps. No result was defined as no diminishment in the pain or aching and no decrease in the size of the lumps. Based on these criteria, 80 cases (62.5%) of the women in this study experienced complete cure; 42 (32.81%) experienced marked improvement; and 6 cases got no result. Thus the total amelioration rate was 95.31%. This formula is based on the principles of rectifying the qi and quickening the blood, transforming phlegm and scattering nodulation.

"The Pattern Discrimination Treatment of 100 Cases of Mammary Hyperplasia" by Fang Jian-ping, *Jiang Su Zhong Yi (Jiang Su Traditional Chinese Medicine)*, #2, 1993, p. 14; BF

This research report describes the treatment of 100 cases of mammary hyperplasia based on treating according to a discrimination of patterns. Of the 100 cases, 97 were female and there were 3 males. Four patients were between the ages of 15-20; 25 between 21-30; 54 between 31-40; and there were 17 cases between 41-50 years of age. Ninety were married and 10 unmarried.

1. Liver depression, qi stagnation pattern (45 cases)

The lumps within these women's breasts were large like date pits or chicken eggs. They also presented with emotional lability, heart vexation, and easy anger, The women's menstruation was not easy and there was premenstrual breast heaviness and discomfort, distention and pain. The tongue coating was thin, white or yellow and the pulse was wiry. The therapeutic principles are to course the liver and resolve depression, move the qi and scatter nodulation.

The formula used was *Xiao Yao San Jia Jian* (Rambling Powder with Additions & Subtractions): vinegar(-fried) Radix Bupleuri (*Cu Chai Hu*) and stir-fried Fructus Gardeniae Jasminoidis (*Chao San Zhi*), 5g @, Radix Albus Paeoniae Lactiflorae (*Bai Shao*), Sclerotium Poriae Cocos (*Fu Ling*), Radix Angelicae Sinensis (*Dang Gui*), Herba Cum Radice Taraxaci Mongolici (*Pu Gong Ying*), Pericarpium Trichosanthis Kirlowii (*Gua Lou Pi*), Pericarpium Viridis Citri Reticulatae (*Qing Pi*), Rhizoma Atractylodis Macrocephalae (*Bai Zhu*), and Semen Citri (*Ju He*), 10g @, Rhizoma Praeparata Zingiberis (*Wei Jiang*) and Radix Glycyrrhizae (*Gan Cao*), 3g @, and processed Squama Manitis Pentadactylis (*Zhi Jia Pian*), 6g.

2. Liver depression, qi vacuity pattern (23 cases)

These women's lumps were divided and scattered or blended into the rest of the tissue and were not easily discernable. They were also movable. Their facial color was sallow white and they had dizziness and vertigo, were exhausted and lacked strength. Their menses were excessive but pale in color, and their tongues were pale with a thin, white coating. Their pulses were soggy and fine. The therapeutic principles for this presentation are to course the liver and scatter nodulation, boost the qi and nourish the blood.

The formula used was *Si Wu Tang Jia Jian* (Four Materials Decoction with Additions & Subtractions): prepared Radix Rehmanniae (*Shu Di*), Radix Angelicae Sinensis (*Dang Gui*), Radix Albus Paeoniae Lactiflorae (*Bai Shao*), Radix Astragali Membranacei (*Huang Qi*), Sclerotium Poriae Cocos (*Fu Ling*), Tuber Curcumae (*Yu Jin*), Herba Cum Radice Taraxaci Mongolici (*Pu Gong Ying*), and Fructus Liquidambaris Taiwaniae (*Lu Lu Tong*), 10g @, Rhizoma Ligustici Wallichii (*Chuan Xiong*) and Cornu Degelatinum Cervi (*Lu Jiao Shuang*), 5g @, vinegar(-fried) Radix Bupleuri (*Cu Chai Hu*), 3g, processed Squama Manitis Pentadactylis (*Zhi Jia Pian*), 6g.

3. Liver depression, phlegm nodulation pattern (18 cases)

These women's lumps were disciform or lobular in shape. Their chests, lateral costal regions, and epigastriums were oppressed and distended accompanied by dizziness, a slightly bitter taste in the mouth, abnormal appetite, clots within their menstrual flow, possible loose stools, a pale tongue with a white, slimy coating, and a slippery pulse. The therapeutic principles in this case are to course the liver and flush phlegm, soften the hard and scatter nodulation.

The formula used was *Lou Feng Fang Tang Jia Jian* (Nidus Vespae Decoction with Additions & Subtractions): Nidus Vespae (*Lou Feng*

Fang), Bulbus Cremastrae (*Shan Ci Gu*), processed Squama Manitis Pentadactylis (*Zhi Jia Pian*), and Radix Bupleuri (*Chai Hu*), 6g @, Tuber Curcumae (*Yu Jin*), Pericarpium Viridis Citri Reticulatae (*Qing Pi*), Bulbus Fritillariae Thunbergii (*Bei Mu*), Folium Citri (*Ju Ye*), 10g @, processed Rhizoma Cyperi Rotundi (*Zhi Xiang Fu*), 12g, and Spica Prunellae Vulgaris (*Xia Gu Cao*), 25g.

4. Qi stagnation, blood stasis pattern (14 cases)

These women's lumps were comparatively firm and like a hard ball in shape. They might also be disciform or lobular. There was aching and pain or pain upon pressure. These lumps had been soft or slippery but had undergone a change. There were clots in these women's menstru-ate and its color was purplish and dark. Their tongues had a purple qi (*i.e.*, color) or purple patches. Their pulses were fine and wiry. The therapeutic principles in this case are to quicken the blood and dispel stasis, soften the hard and scatter nodulation.

The formula used was *Jie Yu Ruan Jian Tang* (Resolve Depression, Soften the Hard Decoction): Radix Angelicae Sinensis (*Quan Dang Gui*), mix-fried Radix Rubrus Paeoniae Lactiflorae (*Chao Chi Shao*), Fructus Tribuli Terrestris (*Bai Ji Li*), Thallus Algae (*Dan Kun Bu*), Herba Sargassii (*Hai Zao*), Cornu Degelatinum Cervi (*Lu Jiao Shuang*), Radix Salviae Miltiorrhizae (*Dan Shen*), and Fructus Crataegi (*Shan Zha*), 10g @, processed Rhizoma Cyperi Rotundi (*Zhi Xiang Fu*), processed Squama Manitis Pentadactylis (*Zhi Jia Pian*), and Tuber Curcumae (*Yu Jin*), 6g @, Rhizoma Ligustici Wallichii (*Chuan Xiong*), Radix Bupleuri (*Chai Hu*), Pericarpium Viridis Citri Reticulatae (*Qing Pi*), and Bulbus Cremastrae (*Shan Ci Gu*), 5g @, and Herba Cum Radice Taraxaci Mongolici (*Pu Gong Ying*), 12g. The above medicinals were administered in decoction internally. At the same time, externally, *Xiao Yan Gao* (Disperse Inflammation Plaster) plus *Ru Kuai San* (Breast Lump Powder, which is composed of Borneolum [*Bing Pian*], Borax [*Yue Shi*], etc.) were applied above the lumps.

The criteria for success using these protocols were as follows: Complete cure was defined as disappearance of the lumps, disappearance of the breast pain, and discontinuance of the medicinals after 3 months. Marked improvement was defined as diminishment of the size of the lumps by half and disappearance of the breast pain. Some improvement was defined as diminishment of the size of the lumps by less than half and reduction in the breast pain. No result was defined as no reduction in the size of the breast lumps.

Thirty-seven cases of liver depression, qi stagnation experienced complete cure; 6, marked improvement; and 2, some improvement. Sixteen cases of liver depression, qi vacuity experienced complete cure; 5, marked improvement; and 2 some improvement. Eleven cases of qi depression, phlegm nodulation experienced complete cure; 5, marked improvement; 1, some improvement; and 1, no result. And 8 cases of qi stagnation, blood stasis experienced complete cure; 3, marked improvement; 1, some improvement; and 2, no result. Therefore, the total number of cures was 72; marked improvement, 19; some improvement, 6; and no result, 3. Thus the total amelioration rate was 97%.

Dysmenorrhea & Endometriosis

"The Treatment of 50 Cases of Dysmenorrhea with _Xiang Cao Tang_ (Cyperus & Leonurus Decoction)" by Yang Yunxia & Zhang Hai-zhen, _He Nan Zhong Yi (Henan Traditional Chinese Medicine)_, #5, 1993, p. 226; BF

Fifty women with dysmenorrhea were treated by the authors with _Xiang Cao Tang_. The oldest of these women was 44 and the youngest was 14. The longest duration of dysmenorrhea was 12 years and the shortest was half a year. Thirty-three cases experienced pain during their menstrual period, 12 after their period, and 5 before. The amount of flow was medium in 27 cases, excessive in 13 cases, and scant in 10 cases. Twenty-six women were unmarried and 24 were married. Forty-seven cases had pain which began 1-2 days before the period and lasted through first day of the period, while 3 cases had abdominal pain after the period. Gynecological exam revealed that 10 cases had a retroverted uterus, 4 had improper uterine development, 15 had abnormal thickening of the body of the uterus and adnexa, 3 had ovarian cysts, and 6 had uterine myomas.

The formula consisted of: Rhizoma Cyperi Rotundi (*Xiang Fu*), 24g, Herba Leonuri Heterophylli (*Yi Mu Cao*), 30g, Caulis Millettiae Seu Spatholobi (*Ji Xue Teng*), 15g, Radix Angelicae Sinensis (*Dang Gui*), 15g, Herba Lycopi Lucidi (*Ze Lan Ye*), 15g, Rhizoma Ligustici Wallichii (*Chuan Xiong*), 6g, Semen Biotae Orientalis (*Bai Zi Ren*), 10g, plus a suitable amount of red (*i.e.*, brown) sugar.

If the amount of the menstruate was excessive and contained clots, Rhizoma Corydalis Yanhusuo (*Yuan Hu*), 15g, calcined Concha Ostreae (*Duan Mu Li*), 20g, and Sanguis Draconis (*Xue Jie*), 2g, were added. If the amount of the menstruate was scanty, Flos Carthami Tinctorii (*Hong Hua*), 15g, and Radix Cyathulae (*Chuan Niu Xi*), 15g, were added. If the uterus was improperly developed, Semen Cuscutae (*Tu Si Zi*), 30g, and Fructus Lycii Chinensis (*Qi Guo*), 15g, were added. If there was pelvic inflammatory disease, Radix Salviae Miltiorrhizae (*Dan Shen*), 30g, and Herba Patriniae Heterophyllae (*Bai Jiang Cao*), 30g, were added. If there were ovarian cysts, Rhizoma Sparganii (*San Leng*), 15g, Rhizoma Curcumae Zedoariae (*Wen Zhu*), 15g, and Herba Dianthi (*Qu Mai*), 15g, were added. If there was uterine myoma, Squama Manitis (*Chuan Shan Jia*), 15g, was added. And if there was pain after the period, Radix Codonopsis Pilosulae (*Dang Shen*), 24g, Folium Artemesiae Argyii (*Ai Ye*), 10g, and Cortex Cinnamomi (*Yuan Rou*), 15g, were added. Beginning 1 week before the onset of the period, 1 *ji* was given per day for 5-7 days.

Using this protocol, all 50 cases were cured. Among those treated, the shortest duration of treatment was 1 menstrual cycle or 7 *ji*. The longest was half a year with 42 *ji*. After treatment the menstruation became normal and the menstrual pain disappeared. Gynecological examinations were also normal.

According to the authors, dysmenorrhea is mostly due to the movement of the qi and blood not being smooth and uninhibited. In this disease, the qi and blood within the *chong* and *ren* and *bao gong* have undergone some (abnormal) change and fail to flow freely. This formula has the ability to both nourish and quicken the blood, transform stagnation and open the channels and vessels. Within this formula, Cyperus enters the qi division (*qi fen*) and is the main medicinal for regulating the menstruation and stopping pain. While Leonurus enters the blood division (*xue fen*) and is the main medicinal for quickening the blood and transforming stasis. These two medicinals thus govern the regulation and rectification of the qi and blood of the *chong* and *ren* and, in terms of dysmenorrhea, are the two main medicinals. Combined with Millettia, Lycopus, Ligusticum, and *Dang Gui*, they quicken the blood, open the channels (or menses), and stop pain. Semen Biotae Orientalis nourishes heart blood and moistens the channels and vessels, while brown sugar guides and opens the hundreds of vessels. Therefore, this formula is really a fine formula for treating dysmenorrhea.

"The Treatment of 40 Cases of Endometriosis by Boosting the Qi and Transforming Stasis" by He Shu-ying, *Si Chuan Zhong Yi (Sichuan Traditional Chinese Medicine)*, #9, 1993, p. 41; BF

All 40 women in this study suffered from endometriosis as diagnosed by gynecological examination and other modern Western medical procedures. Their ages ranged from 24-48 years old, the course of their disease ranged from as short as 1 year to as long as 18 years. Among these 40 women, 25 were infertile. Thirty-one had had previous surgery for ectopic pregnancies, artificial abortions, and other such surgical procedures. Thirty-seven cases experienced occasionally intense abdominal and period pain. Twelve had pain with intercourse. Twenty-eight had pelvic pain. 18 had a heavy, distended, pulling and tugging feeling in their anus.

The formula with which these women were treated consisted of: Radix Codonopsis Pilosulae (*Dang Shen*) and Radix Astragali Membranacei (*Huang Qi*), 20g @, Radix Bupleuri (*Chai Hu*), Pericarpium Citri Reticulatae (*Chen Pi*), Fructus Liquidambaris Taiwaniae (*Lu Lu Tong*), and Rhizoma Corydalis Yanhusuo (*Yan Hu*), 10g @, Rhizoma Cimicifugae (*Sheng Ma*), 6g, raw Radix Rehmanniae (*Sheng Di*), Pollen Typhae (*Pu Huang*), Radix Rubrus Paeoniae Lactiflorae (*Chi Shao*), Gummum Olibani (*Ru*), and Myrrha (*Mo*), 10g @, and Rhizoma Sparganii (*San Leng*) and Rhizoma Curcumae Zedoariae (*E Zhu*), 20g @.

If there was yang vacuity, Radix Praeparatus Aconiti Carmichaeli (*Fu Pian*), 10g, and Cortex Cinnamomi (*Rou Gui*), 6g, were added. If there was severe tugging and pulling aching and pain of the anus, Fructus Foeniculi Vulgaris (*Xiao Hui Xiang*) and Fructus Meliae Toosendan (*Chuan Lian Zi*), 10g @, were added. If there was blood vacuity, Gelatinum Corii Asini (*E Jiao*) and Radix Polygoni Multiflori (*Shou Wu*), 10g @, were added. If there was constipation, raw Radix Et Rhizoma Rhei (*Sheng Jun*), 8g, was added. If the menses was excessive and like a rush, Herba Agrimoniae Pilosae (*Xian He Cao*), 20g, carbonized Radix Scutellariae Baicalensis (*Huang Qin Tan*), 10g, and carbonized Cacumen Biotae (*Ce Bai Tan*), 12g, were added. If there was low back ache, Cortex Eucommiae Ulmoidis (*Du Zhong*), Ramus Loranthi Seu Visci (*Sang Ji Sheng*), and Herba Cistanchis (*Cong Rong*), 10g @, were added. If there were cystic lumps or chocolate cysts, Spina Gleditschiae Chinensis (*Zao Jiao Ci*) and Lignum Sappani (*Su Mu*), 10g @, were added.

Marked improvement was defined as disappearance of the main symptoms and obvious reduction in the nodulations within the pelvis. Some improvement was defined as a reduction in the symptoms and a reduction in the nodulations. Based on these criteria, 33 women experienced marked improvement and 7 conceived afterwards. Four cases experienced some improvement, and 3 cases got no result. Thus the combined amelioration rate was 92.5%.

The author relates this condition primarily to binding of static malign blood. This may be due to either cold congelation or qi stagnation leading to blood stasis. If, however, there is excessive menstrual bleeding like a rush, this is due to insufficient qi and blood. In this case, qi is unable to restrain or to move the blood. Thus qi vacuity changes into blood stagnation. If the qi is vacuous, central qi may fall downward resulting in anal heaviness and distention with tugging and pulling aching and pain. Therefore, in this protocol, Codonopsis, Astragalus, Bupleurum, and Cimicifugae upbear the central qi. These are then combined with medicinals to quicken the blood and transform stasis.

"An Analysis of the Treatment of 35 Cases of Endometriosis Using the Transforming Stasis, Supplementing the Kidneys Method" by Yin Xiu-lan, _Shang Hai Zhong Yi Yao Za Zhi (The Shanghai Journal of Traditional Chinese Medicine & Medicinals)_, #11, 1993, p. 21-2; BF

After defining this condition in Western medical terms, the author says that in Traditional Chinese Medicine it is categorized as menstrual pain (_tong jing_) and conglomerations and concretions (_zheng jia_) and its main associated conditions are period pain, menstrual irregularity, and infertility. The 35 women treated in this study ranged in age from 21-53 years old, with the average being 36.9 years of age. Thirty-four of the cases had dysmenorrhea and menstrual irregularity. Seven women were infertile. Twenty-seven of the women had so-called chocolate ovarian cysts. Gynecologic examination found obviously painful nodulations in 20 cases and 1/3 of the women had retroverted uteri.

This study used a staged protocol involving two different formula. Formula 1 consisted of: raw Radix Astragali Membranacei (*Sheng Huang Qi*) and Radix Salviae Miltiorrhizae (*Dan Shen*), 30g @, Radix Angelicae Sinensis (*Quan Dang Gui*) and Herba Epimedii (*Yin Yang Huo*), 12g @, Radix Rubrus Paeoniae Lactiflorae (*Chi Shao*) and Spica Prunellae Vulgaris (*Xia Gu Cao*), 20g @, Rhizoma Sparganii (*San Leng*), Rhizoma Curcumae Zedoariae (*E Zhu*), and Fructus Ligustri Lucidi (*Nu Zhen Zi*), 10g @, Radix Dipsaci (*Xu Duan*), 15g, raw Radix Et Rhizoma Rhei (*Sheng Da Huang*) and Feces Trogopterori Seu Pteromi (*Wu Ling Zhi*), 6g @, and Sanguis Draconis (*Xue Jie*) 0.3g (ground into powder and swallowed down with the other decocted medicinals).

Formula 2 consisted of: raw Radix Astragali Membranacei (*Sheng Huang Qi*), 30g, Radix Angelicae Sinensis (*Dang Gui*), 9g, Radix Rubrus Paeoniae Lactiflorae (*Chi Shao*), Radix Salviae Miltiorrhizae (*Dan Shen*), Herba Ecliptae Prostratae (*Han Lian Cao*), and raw Radix Rehmanniae (*Sheng Di*), 20g @, raw and stir-fried Pollen Typhae (*Sheng Chao Pu Huang*), 12g @ (wrapped), Radix Rubiae Cordifoliae (*Qian Cao*), Cortex Radicis Lycii (*Di Gu Pi*), and Radix Dipsaci (*Xu Duan*), 15g @, Fructus Ligustri Lucidi (*Nu Zhen Zi*), 10g, Feces Trogopterori Seu Pteromi (*Wu Ling Zhi*), 6g, processed Radix Et Rhizoma Rhei (*Zhi Jun*), 9g, Gummum Olibani (*Ru Xiang*) and Myrrha (*Mo Yao*), 3g @.

Formula 1 was administered from after the cessation of the menstruation till after the next period began, 1 *ji* per day. Then formula 2 was administered. (In other words, formula 2 was administered only during the period itself.) This was continued for from 3-6 months.

If after taking the Sanguis Draconis the patient became nauseous, it was removed and Eupolyphagae Seu Opisthoplatiae (_Di Bie Chong_), 12g, was added. If the menstrual pain was categorized as cold, Eclipta, Agrimonia, Cortex Radicis Lycii, and raw Rehmannia were removed and aged Folium Artemesiae Argyii (_Chen Ai_), 10g, and Fructus Evodiae Rutecarpae (_Wu Zhu Yu_), 3g, were added to warm the channels, scatter cold, and stop pain. If the menstruate was excessive like a downpour and was colored purple and dark with large amounts of blood clots, Ophicalcitum (_Hua Ru Shi_), 30g, was added to dispel stasis and stop pain.

Complete cure consisted of disappearance of the symptoms and the infertile patients becoming pregnant. Marked improvement consisted of disappearance of the symptoms with the cysts or nodules reduced in size by 1/2 or more. Also, those who were infertile conceived. Some improvement meant that the symptoms were stabilized somewhat but the majority of symptoms were not eliminated. And no result meant that there was no change in the condition or it got worse. Based on these criteria, 4 cases or 11.4% were cured, 20 or 57.15 were markedly improved, and 8 or 22.9% got some improvement. Thus, the combined amelioration rate was 91.4%.

The author bases their approach on the sayings that "the kidneys govern reproduction" and that "the _bao tai_ is fastened to the kidneys." Because this condition is often accompanied by infertility, tinnitus, low back and knee soreness and weakness, diminished sexual desire, and other such symptoms corresponding to essence qi deficiency, this condition commonly involves kidney vacuity. Therefore, within this protocol, Epimedium, Dipsacus, and Ligustrum Lucidum warm the kidneys and strengthen yang, enrich and supplement the liver and kidneys, while Astragalus supplements the qi. Then, because many of the other symptoms of endometriosis correspond to blood stasis, these supplementing medicinals are combined with blood-quickening and stasis-transforming ingredients. In this case, kidney vacuity is the root and blood stasis is the branch, and, although transforming stasis is the main principle, it should be accompanied by simultaneous supplementation.

"A Clinical Survey of 40 Cases of Endometriosis" by Zhu Liang-yu, *Shang Hai Zhong Yi Yao Za Zhi (Shanghai Journal of Traditional Chinese Medicine & Medicinals)*, #1, 1994, p. 12-3; BF

This clinical audit discusses the treatment of 40 cases of endometriosis with a combination of retention enemas, injectible TCM medicinals, and laser acupuncture. Of the 40 women, 4 were over 40 years old, 30 were between 30-40, and 6 were less than 30 years old. Twenty-three suffered from primary onset infertility, 14 had previously had children, and 3 were unmarried.

Based on TCM pattern discrimination, these women were divided into 2 large patterns: 1) qi stagnation, blood stasis and 2) cold congelation, blood stasis. The main symptoms of the first pattern included lower abdominal distention and pain with the coming of the period, early, late or erratic periods, a prolonged menses with excessive amounts of blood, as the period went along, increasingly excessive amounts of blood and even more severe abdominal pain, accompanying breast distention and pain, a wiry pulse, a thin, slimy tongue coating, and a pale red or partially red tongue. The main symptoms of the second pattern were lower abdominal chilly pain with the coming of the period, late periods, the movement of the period not easy or smooth, the amount sometimes excessive, as the period went along, increasingly excessive amounts of blood and piercing abdominal pain, accompanying loose stools, a bluish white or darkish tongue with a thin, white coating, and a deep, tight pulse.

The treatment with retention enemas used two different formulas depending on which of these two large patterns the patients were categorized as exhibiting. Patients in the first pattern received

"Endometriosis No. I". This consisted of: Ramulus Cinnamomi (*Chuan Gui Zhi*), 4.5g, Radix Salviae Miltiorrhizae (*Dan Shen*), 9g, Cortex Radicis Moutan (*Dan Pi*), 9g, stir-fried Radix Rubrus Paeoniae Lactiflorae (*Chao Chi Shao*), 9g, Sclerotium Poriae Cocos (*Bai Fu Ling*), 12g, Herba Salviae Chinensis (*Shi Jian Chuan*), 15g, Semen Pruni Persicae (*Tao Ren*), 9g, Radix Linderae Strychnifoliae (*Wu Yao*), 4.5g, Spina Gleditschiae Chinensis (*Zao Jiao Ci*), 12g, processed Gummum Olibani (*Ru Xiang*), 6g, processed Myrrha (*Mo Yao*), 6g, Herba Patriniae Heterophyllae (*Bai Jiang Cao*), 30g, and Rhizoma Curcumae Zedoariae (*E Zhu*), 9g.

Those women who were categorized as belonging to the second large pattern were given "Endometriosis No. II". This consisted of Cortex Cinnamomi (*Rou Gui*), 4.5g, Radix Salviae Miltiorrhizae (*Dan Shen*), 9g, Cortex Radicis Moutan (*Dan Pi*), 9g, stir-fried Radix Rubrus Paeoniae Lactiflorae (*Chi Shao*), 9g, Sclerotium Poriae Cocos (*Bai Fu Ling*), 12g, Herba Salviae Chinensis (*Shi Jian Chuan*), 15g, Fructus Evodiae Rutecarpae (*Dan Zhu Yu*), 4.5g, Radix Saussureae Seu Vladimiriae (*Mu Xiang*), 3g, processed Gummum Olibani (*Ru Xiang*), 6g, processed Myrrha (*Mo Yao*), 6g, Rhizoma Curcumae Zedoariae (*E Zhu*), 9g, Spina Gleditischiae Chinensis (*Zao Jiao Ci*), 12g, and Herba Patriniae Heterophyllae (*Bai Jiang Cao*), 15g.

The above medicinals were soaked in a suitable amount of water and then boiled to obtain 100ml of decoction. This was introduced as a retention enema 1 time per evening, with 10 treatments equalling 1 course. After 3 months, there was 1 follow-up visit.

If there was endometrial nodes in the fornix behind the vagina as revealed by physical examination and obvious poking pain, a vaginal extending instrument (*i.e.*, a vaginal speculum) was inserted into the vagina. Then the area to the rear of the vagina was pressed to find the most painful nodes. These were injected with 4ml of *Fu Fang Dan*

Shen Zhu She Ye (Compound Salvia Injectible Fluid) 1 time every other day, with 10 treatments equalling 1 course.

In addition, He-Ne laser therapy was given to the acupoints *Zi Gong* (M-CA-18), *Guan Yuan* (CV 4), and *a shi* points for bilateral lower abdominal pain and to the *Ba Liao* points for low back pain.

Marked improvement was defined as obvious diminishment of the lumps after treatment, disapperance of symptoms, or conception. Some improvement was defined as diminishment of the lumps or no obvious increase in their size and reduction in symptoms. No result meant that after treatment symptoms were as before or worse. Based on these criteria, 17 patients experienced obvious diminishment in the size of lumps and disappearance of their symptoms. Another 13 conceived. Among these, 6 had suffered from fallopian tube blockage and 7 from ovulatory dysfunction. Nine women experienced some reduction in their lumps and some reduction in their symptoms. While only 1 patient got no result. Thus the total amelioration rate was 97.5%.

According to the author, what is now known as endometriosis is equivalent to what is called *zheng gu*, inveterate concretion in the *Jin Gui ([Essential Formulas from] the Golden Cabinet)*. Based on a combination of this classic and contemporary clinical experience, this condition can be treated by *Gui Zhi Fu Ling Wan Jia Wei* (Cinnamon & Poria Pills with Added Flavors). Within this formula, Ramulus Cinnamomi opens the blood vessels. Poria quiets the righteous qi. Peony regulates the constructive. And Moutan and Persica quicken the blood and transform stasis. Frankincense and Myrrh are added to strengthen this formula's ability to quicken the blood, transform stasis, and stop pain. Large amounts of Patrinia are used to clear heat and disperse inflammation, crack the blood and disperse swelling. Zedoaria, Herba Salviae, and Spina Gleditschiae crack concretions and scatter nodulation. A small amount of Lindera is used for its aromatic, acrid warmth to precipitate and out-thrust the kidney channel and move and scatter the qi.

If cold evils cause cold congelation and blood stasis, Ramulus Cinnamomi is changed to Cortex Cinnamomi. Then Evodia and Saussurea are added to strengthen this formula's ability to warm the channels, quicken the blood, and stop pain. In that case, one flavor, Persica, is subtracted because it is greasy and moist.

Ovarian Cystitis

"The Treatment of 36 Cases of Cystic Inflammation of the Ovaries with *Qing Re Ruan Jian Tang* (Heat-clearing, Softening the Hard Decoction)" by He Ai-bo, *Si Chuan Zhong Yi (Sichuan Traditional Chinese Medicine)*, #9, 1993, p. 44; BF

Most of the women in this clinical audit had cystic inflammation of the ovaries after having artificial abortions and after having been treated clinically with antibiotics. In December of 1991, the author began using a self-composed formula for this condition called *Qing Re Ruan Jian Tang* which they administered on the basis of both a disease discrimination combined with pattern discrimination. The women subsequently treated ranged in age from a low of 20 to a high of 42 years of age, with the average being 31 years old. The longest course of disease was 3 months and the shortest was 1 week. Previously, these women were treated unsuccessfully with not less than 10 doses of antibiotics. If, after 26 doses, there was no reduction in the cysts, they received a laparoscopy. All the women also had ultrasonography. In 3 cases, the cysts were 7 x 5.5cm in size, in 15 cases they were approximately 6.5 x 5.5cm, in 8 cases they were 5.5 x 4.5cm, in 6 cases 3.5 x 2.5cm, and in 4 cases 2.7 x 2.5cm in size.

The formula consisted of: Caulis Sargentodoxae (*Hong Teng*), Ramus Lonicerae (*Ren Dong Teng*), Herba Patriniae Heterophyllae (*Bai Jiang Cao*), Herba Oldenlandiae (*She She Cao*), Spica Prunellae Vulgaris

(*Xia Gu Cao*), Cortex Phellodendri (*Huang Bai*), and Rhizoma Smilacis Glabrae (*Tu Fu Ling*), 15g @, raw Concha Ostreae (*Sheng Mu Li*), Herba Sargassii (*Hai Zao*), and Thallus Algae (*Kun Bu*), 20g @, Pollen Typhae (*Pu Huang*) and Feces Trogopterori Seu Pteromi (*Wu Ling Zhi*), 10g @, and Rhizoma Alismatis (*Ze Xie*) and Semen Plantaginis (*Che Qian Zi*), 10g @.

If there was qi vacuity, Radix Codonopsis Pilosulae (*Dang Shen*), Rhizoma Atractylodis Macrocephalae (*Bai Zhu*), and Radix Astragali Membranacei (*Huang Qi*) were added. If there was kidney vacuity, Radix Dipsaci (*Chuan Duan*), Ramus Loranthi Seu Visci (*Sang Ji Sheng*), and Cortex Eucommiae Ulmoidis (*Du Zhong*) were added. If there was copious white vaginal discharge, Os Sepiae Seu Sepiellae (*Hai Piao Xiao*) and Cortex Cedrelae (*Chun Bai Pi*) were added. If there was spleen and stomach vacuity, parched Fructus Crataegi (*Jiao Shan Zha*) and Endothelium Corneum Gigeriae Galli (*Ji Nei Jin*) were added. If there was a lochia which would not cease, Herba Leonuri Heterophylli (*Yi Mu Cao*) was added. If there was aching and pain in the lower abdomen, Rhizoma Corydalis Yanhusuo (*Yan Hu*) and Fructus Meliae Toosendan (*Chuan Lian Zi*) were added. One week equalled 1 course of treatment.

All the women in this study were cured using this protocol. This meant that blood stopped being discharged from their vaginal tracts, abnormal vaginal discharge was cured, low back and abdominal pain was reduced, and the symptoms disappeared. Ultrasonography showed that the cysts were smaller. Two cases were cured after 1 course of treatment, 4 after 2 courses, 16 after 3 courses, 8 after 4 courses, 5 after 5 courses, and 1 after 10 courses of treatment.

According to the author, this condition mostly occurs after abortions either due to constitutional weakness or insufficient sterilization of the surgical tools. If not treated, it can lead to chronic pelvic inflammatory disease and eventual infertility. Traditional Chinese Medicine categorizes this as conglomerations and concretions and the disease mechanism involves damp heat stasis and gathering. This gathering binds to form a lump. This stasis obstruction in the lower abdomen then results in aching and pain. Because of the stasis and obstruction in the *bao gong*, the *chong* and *ren* suffer detriment and, thus, the menses becomes irregular. Damp heat pouring down results in excessive, white, abnormal vaginal discharge. The principles of treating this condition are to clear heat and transform dampness, soften the hard and scatter nodulation, quicken the blood and transform stasis.

"The Treatment of 26 Cases of Ovarian Cysts by the Methods of Supplementing the Kidneys, Quickening the Blood, and Transforming Stasis" by Liu Li-ling, *Shan Dong Zhong Yi Za Zhi (The Shandong Journal of Traditional Chinese Medicine)*, #3, 1993, p. 23-4; BF

In almost four years, the author has treated 26 cases of ovarian cysts primarily by supplementing the kidneys while simultaneously quickening the blood and transforming stasis. All 26 cases were one-sided, with 11 on the right and 15 on the left. The cysts ranged in size from a large of 10.2 x 9.8cm to a small of 3.2 x 3cm. Among these 26 cases, there were 8 cases of endometrial cysts and 2 cases of teratistic tumorous cysts. Eighteen of these women were married and 8 were not married. All 26 experienced some degree of menstrual irregularity, lower abdominal pain, excessive vaginal discharge. Seven cases had ceased menstruating. All 26 had had ultrasonography.

The medicinals used in this protocol consisted of: Radix Dipsaci (*Chuan Duan*), 15g, Herba Epimedii (*Yin Yang Huo*), 15-30g, Radix Angelicae Sinensis (*Dang Gui*), 10g, Radix Albus Paeoniae Lactiflorae (*Bai Shao*), 10g, Semen Pruni Persicae (*Tao Ren*), 10g, Rhizoma Sparganii (*San Leng*), 10g, Rhizoma Curcumae Zedoariae (*E Zhu*),

111

10g, Semen Cuscutae (*Tu Si Zi*), 10g, and Fluoritum (*Zhi Shi Ying*), 30g. These were decocted in water and administered, 1 *ji* per day.

If vaginal discharge was excessive, Radix Dioscoreae Oppositae (*Shan Yao*) and Herba Cum Radice Taraxaci Mongolici (*Pu Gong Ying*), 15g @, were added. If the menses dribbled and dripped and would not stop, carbonized Radix Sanguisorbae (*Di Yu Tan*), 10g, was added. If there was liver depression and qi stagnation with abdominal pain, Rhizoma Cyperi Rotundi (*Xiang Fu*) and Radix Bupleuri (*Chai Hu*), 10g @, were added.

Complete cure consisted of ultrasonography showing the ovaries on both sides normal with disappearance of lower abdominal pain, low back pain, and menstrual irregularity with no abnormal changes after 3 months. Based on this criteria, 24 women were completely cured. The shortest duration of treatment was 10 *ji* and the longest was 20, with the average being 15 *ji*.

The author defines this condition in TCM as concretions and conglomeration (*zheng jia*) and says that its disease mechanism is mostly kidney vacuity and blood stasis. Since the kidneys govern the *chong* and *ren* and also govern the qi transformation (*qi hua*), kidney vacuity may lead to the *chong* and *ren* losing nourishment and the qi transformation losing its control. In that case, qi, blood, and water fluids may not be able to be moved and transported normally. Thus the functioning of the *ren, du,* and *chong* may become irregular and accumulation results in this condition. As the author notes, the *Ling Shu (Spiritual Axis)* says that stonelike conglomerations in the uterus are due to cold blocking and obstructing the child gate. However, this cold is less often due to external cold and most case are due to kidney yang vacuity with kidney qi being insufficient. Yang vacuity leads to cold and inability of the qi transformation to harmonize and warm the uterus. Thus one sees functional debility with this condition, such as abnormal vaginal discharge, genital frigidity, and low back and knee soreness and weakness. Kidney qi vacuity leads to loss of nourishment

112

of the *chong* and *ren*. In that case, the qi and blood are not able to move and transport normally. Hence, there is stasis obstruction in the lower abdomen which takes the form of cysts.

Infertility

"Five Cases of Infertility Treated by the Artificial Menstrual Cycle Treatment Method with Chinese Medicinals" by Liu Zhong-wei, *Ji Lin Zhong Yi Yao (Jilin Chinese Medicine & Medicinals)*, #4, 1993, p. 27; BF

In 1990, the author treated 5 cases of qi stagnation, blood cold pattern infertility with the so-called artificial menstrual cycle method of treatment. Of these, 4 cases were primary onset infertility and 1 was secondary onset infertility. All the women suffered from menstrual movement abdominal pain, but the color, amount, quality, etc. (of the menstrual blood) was not the same and the degree of their pathology was variable.

Method of Treatment

1. Follicular phase, *i.e.*, postmenstrual phase

During this phase of the menstrual cycle, the treatment principles were to enrich kidneys, fortify the spleen, and nourish the blood as well as to regulate and supplement the *chong* and *ren* in order to promote follicular development.

The formula used consisted of: Radix Dioscoreae Oppositae (*Shan Yao*), 20g, prepared Radix Rehmanniae (*Shu Di*), 20g, Radix Polygoni Multiflori (*Shou Wu*), 25g, Semen Cuscutae (*Tu Si Zi*), 20g, Radix Angelicae Sinensis (*Dang Gui*), 15g, Radix Dipsaci (*Chuan Duan*), 10g, Herba Cistanchis (*Rou Cong Rong*), 10g, and Placenta Hominis

(*Zi He Che*), 30g (added at the end after the cooking). These were decocted in water and taken; 1 day, 2 doses.

2. Ovulatory phase, *i.e.*, intermenstrual phase

During this phase, the treatment principles were to supplement the kidneys, warm, and free the flow, quicken the blood and transform stasis so as to promote unimpeded ovulation.

The formula used consisted of: Radix Angelicae Sinensis (*Dang Gui*), 20g, Rhizoma Ligustici Wallichii (*Chuan Xiong*), 15g, Herba Lycopi Lucidi (*Ze Lan*), 15g, prepared Radix Rehmanniae (*Shu Di*), 15g, Rhizoma Cyperi Rotundi (*Xiang Fu*), 10g, Flos Carthami Tinctorii (*Hong Hua*), 5g, Semen Pruni Persicae (*Tao Ren*), 5g, Radix Rubrus Paeoniae Lactiflorae (*Chi Shao*), 10g, Fructus Foeniculi Vulgaris (*Hui Xiang*), 5g, Folium Artemesiae Argyii (*Ai Ye*), 10g, and Herba Photiniae Serrulatae (*Shi Nan Ye*), 15g. If the patient continues to be infertile, it is alright to add Herba Epimedii (*Xian Ling*), Radix Angelicae (*Bai Zhi*), Fructus Liquidambaris Taiwaniae (*Lu Lu Tong*), etc.

3. Luteal phase, *i.e.*, premenstrual phase

During this phase, the treatment principles were to warm the kidneys and warm the uterus so as to promote normalcy of hormonal secretions.

The formula used consisted of: Prepared Radix Rehmanniae (*Shu Di*), 20g, Radix Angelicae Sinensis (*Dang Gui*), 20g, Radix Dioscoreae Oppositae (*Shan Yao*), 15g, Sclerotium Poriae Cocoris (*Fu Ling*), 15g, Radix Codonopsis Pilosulae (*Dang Shen*), 15g, Fructus Lycii Chinensis (*Gou Qi Zi*), 20g, Folium Artemesiae Argyii (*Ai Ye*), 10g, Ramulus Cinnamomi (*Gui Zhi*), 10g, Radix Morindae Officinalis (*Ba Ji*), 10g, and Placenta Hominis (*Zi He Che*), 30g (added at the end after the cooking). These were decocted in water and taken; 1 day, 2 doses.

4. Menstrual Phase

The treatment principles used during this phase were to quicken the blood and regulate the menses.

The formula used consisted of: Radix Angelicae (*Dang Gui*), 15g, Radix Rubrus Paeoniae Lactiflorae (*Chi Shao*), 15g, Herba Leonuri Heterophylli (*Yi Mu Cao*), 20g, Radix Salviae Miltiorrhizae (*Dan Shen*), 10g, Rhizoma Cyperi Rotundi (*Xiang Fu*), 10g, Herba Lycopi Lucidi (*Ze Lan*), 10g, and Sclerotium Poriae Cocos (*Fu Ling*), 10g

Using the above protocol, all 5 cases were cured. Three conceived after 2 whole cycles of treatment, and the other 2 became pregnant after 3 whole cycles of treatment.

Case history: The woman was 28 years old and had been married for 3 years without getting pregnant. Gynecological examination revealed no obvious pathological changes and her serum hormones were normal. TCM examination revealed that her menses was typically three days late. When the period came there was lower abdominal chilly pain. The amount of flow was scant and its color was purple and dark with blood clots. Abnormal vaginal discharge was excessive. There was also breast distention and pain and her pulse was deep and thready. She was diagnosed as qi stagnation, blood cold pattern infertility. She was administered the above protocol, 1 formula (*i.e.*, packet) of medicinals per day. After one whole cycle the abdominal pain with her period was already eliminated. She conceived during the second cycle of treatment. Thus clinically, the treatment was a cure.

"Liu Hong-xiang's Experience in Treating Ovarian Function Impediment" by Wang Guang-hui, *Shan Dong Zhong Yi Za Zhi (The Shandong Journal of Traditional Chinese Medicine)*, #4, 1993, p. 43; BF

This is another report on treating infertility using the artificial menstrual cycle treatment method. Like many other modern TCM infertility protocols it is based on the idea that "the *tian gui* is rooted in the kidneys." As in the above infertility protocol, this one also uses four separate formulas during each of the phases of the menstrual cycle. However, in this protocol, Dr. Wang divides the luteal phase into the luteal transformative phase and the premenstruum.

1. Follicular phase, *i.e.*, postmenstrual phase

Based on the principles of enriching kidney yin and fulfilling essence and blood during this phase, the following formula was given from days 4-11: prepared Radix Rehmanniae (*Shu Di*), Sclerotium Poriae Cocos (*Fu Ling*), Rhizoma Alismatis (*Ze Xie*), Radix Angelicae Sinensis (*Dang Gui*), Radix Dipsaci (*Xu Duan*), and Herba Epimedii (*Xian Ling Pi*), 12g each, Fructus Lycii Chinensis (*Gou Qi*), Ramus Loranthi Seu Visci (*Ji Sheng*), and Fluoritum (*Zi Shi Ying*), 15g each, Radix Dioscoreae Oppositae (*Shan Yao*), 20 g, and Fructus Corni (*Shan Zhu Rou*), 10g. These were decocted in water, each day 1 *ji*.

If there is simultaneous blood vacuity, this was combined with *Si Wu Tang* (Four Materials Decoction) and prepared Radix Rehmanniae was changed to raw Radix Rehmanniae (*Sheng Di*). If there was yin vacuity with yang effulgence, Radix Scrophulariae Ningpoensis (*Xuan Shen*) and Rhizoma Anemarrhenae (*Zhi Mu*) were added. If there was vexatious heat in the five hearts, *Er Zhi Wan* (Two Ultimates Pills, *i.e.*, Herba Ecliptae Prostratae [*Han Lian Cao*] and Fructus Ligustri Lucidi [*Nu Zhen Zi*]) were added. And if there was heart vexation and lack of sleep, Semen Zizyphi Spinosae (*Suan Zao Ren*) was added.

2. Ovulatory phase, *i.e.*, intermenstrual phase

The treatment principles given in this report for this phase in the menstrual cycle are to boost the qi and quicken the blood, supplement the kidneys and free the flow of yang. This phase lasts from the 12-15 days of the cycle. The formula used consisted of: Radix Astragali Membranacei (*Huang Qi*), Radix Albus Paeoniae Lactiflorae (*Bai Shao*), and Rhizoma Dioscoreae Hypoglaucae (*Bi Xie)*, 20g each, Radix Dipsaci (*Xu Duan*), Herba Epimedii (*Xian Ling Pi*), prepared Radix Rehmanniae (*Shu Di*), Ramus Loranthi Seu Visci (*Ji Sheng*), Fluoritum (*Zi Shi Ying*), and Radix Angelicae Sinensis (*Dang Gui*), 15g each, Ramulus Cinnamomi (*Gui Zhi*), 12g, and Rhizoma Ligustici Wallichii (*Chuan Xiong*), 10g. These were decocted in water and taken, 1 *ji* per day.

If there was diminished sex drive, Rhizoma Curculiginis Orchoidis (*Xian Mao*), Herba Cistanchis (*Rou Cong Rong*), and Radix Morindae Officinalis (*Ba Ji Tian*) were added, and the amount of Fluoritum was increased and the amount of Epimedium doubled. If there was intermenstrual bleeding, it was not necessarily treated if the amount was small but was treated if the amount was more. If it was categorized as kidney yin deficiency and vacuity, evil heat arising within, the above was combined with *Er Di Qin Shao Tang* (Two Rehmannias, Scutellaria, & Peony Decoction) which consists of: Radix Rehmanniae (*Sheng Di*), Radix Sanguisorbae (*Di Yu*), Radix Scutellariae Baicalensis (*Huang Qin*), and Radix Albus Paeoniae Lactiflorae (*Bai Shao*). If the bleeding was due to damp heat, the above formula was combined with *Jia Wei San Miao San* (Added Flavors Three Marvels Pills, *i.e.*, Rhizoma Atractylodis [*Cang Zhu*], Cortex Phellodendri [*Huang Bai*], Radix Achyranthis Bidentatae [*Niu Xi*], Rhizoma Smilacis Glabrae [*Tu Fu Ling*], Sclerotium Poriae Cocos [*Fu Ling*], and Semen Plantaginis [*Che Qian Zi*]). If liver depression had transformed into fire, the above formula was combined with *Dan Zhi Xiao Yao San* (Moutan & Gardenia Rambling Powder). If the blood was excessive and contained clots with piercing lower abdominal pain, the above formula was combined with *Hua Yu Zhi Lou Tang* (Transform Stasis, Stop Leakage Decoction, *i.e.*, Radix Angelicae Sinensis [*Dang Gui*], Rhizoma Ligustici Wallichii [*Chuan Xiong*], Fructus Crataegi [*Shan Zha*], stir-fried Pollen Typhae [*Pu Huang*], and Feces Trogopterori Seu Pteromi [*Wu Ling Zhi*]). And if there was stasis and heat, Radix Et Rhizoma Rhei (*Da Huang*) was added.

3. Luteal body transformation phase

This phase lasts from days 16-23. During it, the principles of treatment were to regulate the liver and harmonize the spleen aided by supplementing the kidneys and boosting the qi. The formula used consisted of: Radix Angelicae Sinensis (*Dang Gui*), Radix Albus Et Rubrus Paeoniae Lactiflorae (*Chi Bai Shao*), Rhizoma Alismatis (*Ze Xie*), Sclerotium Poriae Cocos (*Fu Ling*), Herba Lycopi Lucidi (*Ze Lan*), Herba Cistanchis (*Rou Cong Rong*), Herba Epimedii (*Xian Ling Pi*), and Semen Cuscutae (*Tu Si Zi*), 15g each, Rhizoma Ligustici Wallichii (*Chuan Xiong*), 10g, Rhizoma Atractylodis Macrocephalae (*Bai Zhu*), Rhizoma Cyperi Rotundi (*Xiang Fu*), and Ramulus Cinnamomi (*Gui Zhi*), 12g each, Rhizoma Dioscoreae Hypoglaucae (*Bie Xie*) and Ramus Loranthi Seu Visci (*Ji Sheng*), 30g each, and processed Radix Praeparatus Aconiti Carmichaeli (*Zhi Fu Zi*), 6g. These were decocted in water, 1 *ji* per day.

If there was torpid intake and abdominal distention, the above was combined with *Shi Pi Yin* (Bolster the Spleen Decoction). If a fat patient had phlegm, Rhizoma Pinelliae Ternatae (*Fa Ban Xia*) and Succus Bambusae (*Zhu Li*) were added. If the body was thin and vacuity heat had arisen within, Herba Artemesiae Apiaceae (*Qing Hao*), Rhizoma Anemarrhenae (*Zhi Mu*), and Plastrum Testudinis (*Gui Ban*) were added. If there was emotional irritation with lower abdominal pain and diarrhea, the above was combined with *Tong Xie Yao Fang* (Essential Formula for Painful Diarrhea). If there was fifth watch diarrhea (*i.e.*, daybreak diarrhea), the above formula was combined with *Si Shen Wan* (Four Spirits Pills).

4. Premenstrual phase

This phase lasts from the 24-28 days. During it, yin and yang are undergoing transformation and commonly the liver and kidneys are insufficient. Therefore, the treatment principles were to warm and supplement kidney yang, quicken the blood and regulate the menses. The formula used consisted of: Fructus Evodiae Rutecarpae (*Wu Zhu Yu*), Ramulus Cinnamomi (*Gui Zhi*), dry Rhizoma Zingiberis (*Gan Jiang*), Rhizoma Ligustici Wallichii (*Chuan Xiong*), Tuber Ophiopogonis Japonicae (*Mai Dong*), and mix-fried Radix Glycyrrhizae (*Gan Cao*), 10g each, Radix Angelicae Sinensis (*Dang Gui*), Radix Albus Paeoniae Lactiflorae (*Bai Shao*), and Radix Codonopsis Pilosulae (*Dang Shen*), 15g each, and Semen Cuscutae (*Tu Si Zi*), 12g, 1 *ji* per day.

If there was premenstrual breast distention and pain, Fructus Tricho-santhis Kirlowii (*Gua Lou*), Fructus Citri Sacrodactyli (*Fo Shou*), Semen Citri (*Ju He*), Radix Saussureae Seu Vladimiriae (*Mu Xiang*), and Tuber Curcumae (*Yu Jin*) were added. If there was distention and pain with the period, Rhizoma Corydalis Yanhusuo (*Yan Hu Suo*), Radix Linderae Strychnifoliae (*Wu Yao*), Fructus Meliae Toosendanis (*Chuan Lian Zi*), and Rhizoma Cyperi Rotundi (*Xiang Fu*) were added. If there was a feeling of lower abdominal chill with the four limbs not warm, Fructus Foeniculi Vulgaris (*Xiao Hui Xiang*) and Radix Linderae Strychnifoliae (*Wu Yao*) were added. If cold and stasis appeared simultaneously, the above formula was combined with *Shao Fu Zhu Yu Tang* (Lower Abdomen Dispel Stasis Decoction). If there were conglomerations and concretions in the uterus (*i.e.*, uterine masses), the above formula was combined with *Gui Zhi Fu Ling Wan* (Cinnamon & Poria Pills).

"The Treatment of 76 Cases of Fallopian Tube Blockage Infertility with *Shu Tong Tang* (Soothing & Opening Decoction)" by Wang Hong-bo *et al., Si Chuan Zhong Yi (Sichuan Traditional Chinese Medicine)*, #7, 1993, p. 41; BF

This clinical audit reports on 76 women suffering from infertility due to fallopian tube blockage who were treated with both internally administered decoctions and externally applied poultices. Among the 76 women, 53 had fallopian tube blockage due to inflammation. Twelve women had obstructional blockage. Nine women had tubercular blockage. And 2 women had congenital blockage of their tubes.

Based on the assumption that fallopian tube blockage is a stasis condition due either to liver qi and depression binding or cold dampness obstructing and stagnating with consequent obstruction of the *bao mai*, all the women in this study were given *Shu Tong Tang* internally. This consisted of: Radix Salviae Miltiorrhizae (*Dan Shen*), Rhizoma Cyperi Rotundi (*Xiang Fu*), and Radix Albus Paeoniae Lactiflorae (*Bai Shao*), 15g @, Radix Bupleuri (*Chai Hu*), Fructus Citri Seu Ponciri (*Zhi Ke*), Rhizoma Ligustici Wallichii (*Chuan Xiong*), Gummum Olibani (*Ru Xiang*), Myrrha (*Mo Yao*), Fructus Meliae Toosendan (*Chuan Lian Zi*), Fructus Liquidambaris Taiwaniae (*Lu Lu Tong*), Semen Pruni Persicae (*Tao Ren*), and Squama Manitis (*Chuan Shan Jia*), 10g @, and Folium Citri (*Ju Ye*), 12g.

If the patient experienced menstrual irregularity, luteal phase defect, or dysmenorrhea, treatment was modified based on a discrimination of patterns. For instance, if there was concomitant kidney yin vacuity, during the postmenstrual phase (*i.e.*, days 4-11 in the cycle), Fructus Ligustri Lucidi (*Nu Zhen Zi*), Fructus Lycii Chinensis (*Gou Qi Zi*), Herba Ecliptae Prostratae (*Han Lian Cao*), Semen Cuscutae (*Tu Si Zi*), Radix Dioscoreae Oppositae (*Huai Shan Yao*), 30g @, and other such enriching and supplementing liver and kidney medicinals were added. If there was kidney yang vacuity, Herba Epimedii (*Xian Ling Pi*) and Rhizoma Curculiginis Orchoidis (*Xian Mao*), 10g @, Placenta

Hominis (*Zi He Che*), 15g, and other such warming and supplementing kidney yang medicinals were added which are beneficial for strengthening corpus luteal function. If the spleen and kidneys were vacuous, Radix Codonopsis Pilosulae (*Dang Shen*), Radix Dioscoreae Oppositae (*Shan Yao*), and Radix Astragali Membranacei (*Huang Qi*), 30g @, were added.

Externally, *Xiao Yu San* (Disperse Stasis Powder, a formula from the Beijing College of TCM) was applied. This consisted of: Herba Tougucao (*Tou Gu Cao*), 200g, Hirudo Seu Whitmaniae (*Shui Zhi*), Tabanus (*Meng Chong*), Radix Et Rhizoma Rhèi (*Da Huang*), Ramulus Cinnamomi (*Gui Zhi*), and Radix Praeparatus Aconiti Carmichaeli (*Fu Zi*), 10g @, Thallus Algae (*Kun Bu*), 20g, Caulis Sargentodoxae (*Hong Teng*), Radix Rubrus Paeoniae Lactiflorae (*Chi Shao*), and Cortex Radicis Moutan (*Dan Pi*), 15g @, and Semen Arecae Catechu (*Bing Lang*), 12g. These medicinals were put in a cloth bag and steamed thoroughly. After they were hot, they were then applied to the lower abdomen 1 time per day for 20-30 minutes each time. One bag of herbs can be used for 5 days before changing.

According to the authors, the main medicinals, *i.e.*, Bupleurum, Peony, Citrus, and Cyperus, course the liver and rectify the qi. Persica and Salvia quicken the blood, transform stasis, and open the channels. Squama Manitis and Fructus Liquidambaris quicken the blood and break stasis, move the qi and open the network vessels. All these medicinals combined have the effect of coursing the liver and rectifying the qi, quickening the blood and opening the network vessels, warming the channels and scattering cold, and boosting the qi and nourishing the blood.

After 1 course of treatment with this protocol, 70 cases got an effect. Of these, 43 or 56.58% conceived. Six cases or 7.81% got no result. Thus the total amelioration rate was 92.19%.

Post-abortion Sequelae

"The Pattern Discrimination Treatment of Bleeding After Surgical Abortion" by Ou Xiao-qing, *Si Chuan Zhong Yi (Sichuan Traditional Chinese Medicine)*, #7, 1993, p. 42; BF

This is a report on the author's treatment of three cases of bleeding after surgical abortion. The author states that bleeding after surgery is a commonly seen condition and goes on to suggest that it should be treated on the basis of a TCM discrimination of patterns. They then go on to give three case histories of the treatment of post-abortion bleeding associated with three different patterns.

1. Static blood not expelled, new blood not engendered

The patient was a 23 year old woman who had had an abortion a half month previously and had vaginal bleeding which was moderate in amount, purplish red in color, and contained blood clots. She also had lower abdominal piercing pain which resisted pressure. When clots were expelled, the pain diminished. She did not have any fever and her appetite and excretions were normal. Her tongue was pale red with purple spots and a thin, white coating. Her pulse was fine.

According to TCM, the metal knife had caused damage and her *bao mai* had suffered injury. Thus malign blood had remained inside, and this static blood had not been expelled. Therefore, fresh or new blood was not able to enter or gather in the channels. For this, treatment should quicken the blood and dispel stasis while leading the blood to gather in the channels. The prescription consisted of: Radix Angelicae Sinensis (*Dang Gui*), Rhizoma Ligustici Wallichii (*Chuan Xiong*), Feces Trogopterori Seu Pteromi (*Wu Ling Zhi*), Semen Pruni Persicae (*Tao Ren*), and blackened Rhizoma Zingiberis (*Hei Jiang*), 10g @, mix-fried Radix Glycyrrhizae (*Zhi Gan Cao*), 6g, Radix Pseudoginseng (_Shen San Qi_, taken separately), 3g, and Herba Leonuri Heterophylli (_Yi Mu Cao_), 20g. These were decocted in water and taken, 1 _ji_ per day divided in 2 doses. After 3 _ji_ a large date-like purplish black clot was discharged from the vaginal tract. Subsequent to that, the blood flow diminished and then stopped.

2. Bodily vacuity (due to) many births, kidney qi loses (its ability) to secure

The patient was a 38 year old woman. Ten days after an abortion, she experienced vaginal bleeding which would not stop. Its amount was medium, its color was red, and there were no blood clots. The patient's low back was sore and felt like it was going to break. There was also urgent abdominal pain and movement caused her to be dizzy and to sweat. Her appetite was still ok and her excretions were still regular. Her tongue was pale red with a thin, white coating, and her pulse was wiry and fine.

In her case, numerous abortions had resulted in kidney vacuity and her _bao mai_ losing its ability to secure (or consolidate). Qi vacuity caused the blood not to be able to be absorbed or restrained and thus blood was not able to abide in the channels. Treatment required supplementing the kidneys and boosting the qi and securing and restraining the _bao mai_. The prescription consisted of: Radix Codonopsis Pilosulae (_Dang Shen_), 15g, Radix Astragali Membranacei (_Huang Qi_), 20g, Cortex Eucommiae Ulmoidis (_Du Zhong_), Ramus Loranthi Seu Visci (_Sang Ji Sheng_), Radix Angelicae Sinensis (_Dang Gui_), Rhizoma Ligustici Wallichii (_Chuan Xiong_), Semen Pruni Persicae (_Tao Ren_), blackened Rhizoma Zingiberis (_Hei Jiang_), carbonized Rhizoma Dryopteridis Seu Blechni (_Guan Zhong_), and Herba Leonuri Hetero-phylli (_Yi Mu Cao_), 10g @, mix-fried Radix Glycyrrhizae (_Zhi Gan Cao_), 5g, and Rhizoma Cimicifugae (_Sheng Ma_), 3g. These were decocted and taken as usual.

After 4 *ji*, the blood flowing from the vaginal tract had stopped. However, there was still low back soreness and dizziness. Therefore, Persica, *Guan Zhong*, and Leonurus were subtracted from the original formula, and stir-fried Rhizoma Atractylodis Macrocephalae (*Bai Zhu*) and Sclerotium Poriae Cocos (*Fu Ling*), 10g @, were added in order to strengthen the spleen and boost the qi. After 5 more *ji*, the patient's condition had obviously returned to normal.

3. Post-surgical lack of discipline, invasion of external evils

The patient was a 21 year old woman who 1 week after an abortion resumed sexual activity. This resulted in copious, dark purplish blood which contained clots and smelled offensive exiting from her vaginal tract. There was abdominal pain which resisted pressure, no fever, normal appetite, and regular excretions. Her tongue was red with a thin, yellow coating, and her pulse was wiry and rapid. In this case, resumption of sexual activity too soon after abortion had resulted in infection. Evils had entered her *bao gong* and stasis and heat had become mutually bound. The appropriate treatment was to clear heat and resolve toxins, quicken the blood and dispel stasis. The prescription consisted of: Caulis Sargentodoxae (*Hong Teng*), Herba Patriniae Heterophyllae (*Bai Jiang Cao*), and Herba Cum Radice Taraxaci Mongolici (*Pu Gong Ying*), 20g @, Radix Angelicae Sinensis (*Dang Gui*), Rhizoma Ligustici Wallichii (*Chuan Xiong*), Semen Pruni Persicae (*Tao Ren*), Herba Leonuri Heterophylli (*Yi Mu Cao*), Cortex Radicis Moutan (*Dan Pi*), and Radix Salviae Miltiorrhizae (*Dan Shen*), 10g @, and raw Radix Glycyrrhizae (*Sheng Gan Cao*), 6g. These were decocted as usual and taken. After 5 *ji*, the vaginal tract bleeding was diminished and the abdominal pain was lessened. After another 4 *ji* of the above formula, the bleeding stopped and the disease was cured.

"The Treatment of 80 Cases of Post-surgical Abortion Excessive Menstruation with *Gu Jing Wan* (Secure the Menses Pills)" by Mi Yang, *Hu Bei Zhong Yi Za Zhi (The Hubei Journal of Traditional Chinese Medicine)*, #2, 1993, p. 9; BF

From 1981-1991, the author treated 80 cases of excessively heavy periods with *Gu Jing Wan* in women who had had artificial surgical abortions. The patients ranged in age from 22-39 years old, with 24 being between 22-25, 45 between 26-35, and 11 between 36-39 years of age. Forty-two women were categorized as suffering from functional heavy periods. Twenty women's heavy periods were considered due to retaining parts of the embryo. And 18 cases were due to endometriosis.

The medicinals were administered as a decoction (despite the name of the formula). They consisted of: mix-fried Plastrum Testudinis (*Zhi Gui Ban*), 10g, Radix Albus Paeoniae Lactiflorae (*Bai Shao*), 12g, carbonized Radix Scutellariae Baicalensis (*Huang Qin Tan*), 30g, Cortex Cedrelae (*Chun Gen Pi*), Rhizoma Cyperi Rotundi (*Xiang Fu*), and Cortex Phellodendri (*Huang Bai*), 9g @. These were decocted in 500ml of water and taken in 2 divided doses, 1 *ji* per day.

If, after abortion, the period was excessive in amount and dribbled and dripped without cease, if its color was purplish red and contained clots, if there was abdominal pain which disliked pressure, and if there was excessive, abnormal vaginal discharge with an offensive odor, a red tongue with yellow coating, and a deep, rapid pulse, stir-fried Feces Trogopterori Seu Pteromi (*Chao Wu Ling Zhi*), 15g, carbonized Pollen Typhae (*Pu Huang Tan*), 10g, and blast-fried, carbonized Rhizoma Zingiberis (*Pao Jiang Tan*), 9g, were added to the original formula.

If, after abortion, the period was excessive, purplish red in color, was pasty in consistency and had an offensive odor, if there was vexation and agitation, a thirsty mouth, pain within the abdomen, cold and heat rising up and then hiding, the stools dry and bound, reddish urine, a red tongue with a yellow coating, and a rapid, forceful pulse, then Flos Lonicerae Japonicae (*Yin Hua*), Fructus Forsythiae Suspensae (*Lian Qiao*), and Herba Patriniae Heterophyllae (*Bai Jiang Cao*), 30g @, and carbonized Cortex Radicis Moutan (*Dan Pi Tan*) and carbonized Radix Rubiae Cordifoliae (*Qian Cao Tan*), 15g @ were added to the original formula.

If, after abortion, the menses was excessive in amount but its color was pale red and watery accompanied by heart palpitations, shortness of breath, a faded, yellow facial color, fatigue, lack of strength, a pale tongue with a thin, white coating, and a fine, weak pulse, Radix Astragali Membranacei (*Huang Qi*), 15g, Radix Codonopsis Pilosulae (*Dang Shen*), Rhizoma Atractylodis Macrocephalae (*Bai Zhu*), and Gelatinum Corii Asini (*E Jiao,* dissolved at the end), 10g @, and Os Sepiae Seu Sepiellae (*Wu Zei Gu*), 15g, were added to the original formula.

If, after abortion, the period was sometimes excessive and sometimes scanty, dribbled and dripped without stopping, and was accompanied by chest and lateral costal bitterness (*i.e.,* pain) and oppression, belching, acid eructation, sighing, diminished appetite, emotional depression, premenstrual breast distention and pain, a red tongue with a yellow coating, and a wiry pulse, Radix Bupleuri (*Chai Hu*), Fructus Gardeniae Jasminoidis (*Shan Zhi Zi*), Radix Angelicae Sinensis (*Dang Gui*), and Fructus Citri Sacrodactylis (*Fo Shou*), 9g @, were added to the original formula.

And if, after abortion, the menses came bright red, dribbled and dripped without ceasing, and were accompanied by heart vexation, confused thoughts, dizziness, tinnitus, low back and knee soreness and weakness, a dry mouth and throat, a red tongue with yellow coating, and a fine, rapid pulse, Herba Ecliptae Prostratae (*Han Lian Cao*), Fructus Ligustri Lucidi (*Nu Zhen Zi*), and Fructus Corni Officinalis (*Shan Yu Rou*), 9g @, and carbonized raw Radix Rehmanniae (*Sheng*

Di Tan), 15g, were added to the original formula.

Complete cure consisted of the menstrual amount, color, and consistency returning to normal with no recurrence within 3 months of stopping the medicinals. Fair improvement consisted of the color, amount, and consistency of the periods returning to normal, but within 3 months after stopping these medicinals, the periods became excessive again. No result meant that there was no change in the patient's condition after 3 whole months of treatment. Based on these criteria, 42 cases were cured, 30 cases were somewhat improved, and 8 cases got no result. Thus the total amelioration rate was 90%. The course of treatment lasted between 10-60 days, with the average being 20-30 days.

Dr. Mi starts their discussion of this protocol by quoting the *Fu Ren Mi Ke (Women's Department Secrets),* "If the menstrual water comes on supremely excessive, no matter whether (the woman is) fat or skinny, this pertains to heat." Therefore, according to Dr. Mi, this formula has the functions of clearing heat, cooling the blood, and securing and restraining the *chong* and *ren.* However, it can be modified to also treat concomitant blood stasis, spleen vacuity, liver depression, kidney vacuity by adding medicinals which transform stasis, boost the qi, course the liver, and supplement the kidneys.

"The Treatment of 70 Cases of Post-dilation Menstrual Irregularity by the Methods of Boosting the Qi and Transforming Stasis" by Zhu Hong-yun, *Shang Hai Zhong Yi Yao Za Zhi (The Shanghai Journal of Traditional Chinese Medicine & Medicinals),* #4, 1993, p. 14-5; BF

Post-dilation menstrual irregularity is one of the commonly seen diseases in gynecology departments. The menses may be excessive in amount, early, or prolonged, or there may be midcycle bleeding or other such irregularities. From 1988-1990, the author treated 70 cases of this disease using the methods of boosting the qi and transforming stasis. The ages of these women ranged from 22-45. The duration of their condition had lasted from as short as 3 months to as long as 2 years. Thirty cases or 42.9% were associated with dilation performed during abortions. Twenty-nine cases experienced excessively heavy periods, 9 cases early periods, 16 cases prolonged periods, and 16 cases intermenstrual bleeding. Many of these women also suffered from dizziness, heart palpitations, lack of strength, shortness of breath, low back soreness and pain, etc. These women had previously been treated by Western medicine antibiotics and hemostatics. While using the protocol described herein, they were instructed to stop using any other Western or Chinese medicinals.

Further, all the women in this study had had (cervical) dilations. Prior to these dilations, their periods had been normal. Now their periods were either coming 7 or more days early or were lasting more than 7 days. The amount of blood lost during any one period was more than 80ml. Or they had blood exiting from their external vaginal tracts during their menstrual cycle at irregular times.

The medicinals given consisted of: Radix Codonopsis Pilosulae (*Dang Shen*), Radix Pseudostellariae (*Tai Zi Shen*), and Radix Astragali Membranacei (*Huang Qi*), 30g @, Rhizoma Atractylodis Macrocephalae (*Bai Zhu*), Sclerotium Poriae Cocos (*Fu Ling*), Radix Rehmanniae (*Di Huang*), Radix Angelicae Sinensis (*Dang Gui*), Fructus Corni Officinalis (*Shan Yu Rou*), Radix Dipsaci (*Chuan Xu Rou*), and Rhizoma Cyperi Rotundi (*Xiang Fu*), 12g @, Shi Xiao San (Loss of Smile Powder, *i.e.*, Feces Trogopterori Seu Pteromi [*Wu Ling Zhi*] & Pollen Typhae [*Pu Huang*], wrapped separately), carbonized Rhizoma Dryopteridis Seu Blechni (*Guan Zhong Tan*), 15g, Pulvis Radicis Pseudoginseng (*San Qi Fen*), and Radix Glycyrrhizae (*Gan Cao*), 6g. The above medicinals, excluding the Pseudoginseng which was taken separately, were decocted in water and taken in 3 divided doses per day, 1 *ji* per day. Each time the menses came, 5 *ji* were administered which comprised 1 course of treatment. This was repeated in succession for 2 courses.

Complete cure consisted of the period returning to normal after discontinuing these medicinals. Each period, the amount of blood lost was between 50-80ml. There was no recurrence within 3 months of stopping the maoist medicinals. They were also able to retain an IUD within their uterus for more than 1 year afterwards. Marked improvement consisted of these women's periods and menstrual cycles returning to normal after stopping this protocol. Each month they lost only between 50-80ml of blood. However, the condition recurred within 3 months of stopping treatment. Good improvement consisted of the amount of menstruate returning to normal while taking these medicinals. Their menstrual cycles remained short however, even though the amount of blood lost was reduced overall. No result meant there was no change in their clinical presentation. Based on these criteria, 56 women were cured, 7 markedly improved, 3 experienced good improvement, and 4 experienced no result. Thus the cure rate was 80% and the total amelioration rate was 94.3%.

According to Dr. Zhu, post-dilation excessive menstrual bleeding is categorized as a menstrual disease (*yue jing bing*) in TCM. It is usually seen in women with habitually insufficient bodies (*i.e.*, constitutions) who have been dilated during artificial surgical abortions. In such women, their righteous qi is vacuous and weak and this is the cause of the onset of this disease. Clinically, these women's signs and symptoms include loss of regularity of the menses, an ashen white facial color, fatigued limbs and exhausted spirit, shortness of breath, sluggish speech, heart palpitations, dizziness, low back and knee soreness and weakness, diminished appetite, a pale tongue, and a fine pulse as well as other symptoms of righteous qi insufficiency. Western medicines, such as antibiotics and hemostatics, are, more often than not, ineffective, while Chinese medicinals are able to treat this condition by supplementing insufficiency.

The disease mechanism of post-dilation menstrual irregularity is qi vacuity and blood stasis with loss of regularity of the *chong* and *ren*. If there is repeated loss of blood, the qi follows the blood consumption. The qi is not able to restrain the blood and so even more blood is lost. This blood loss then consumes the qi and these two conditions mutually exacerbate each other. When qi and blood both become vacuous and deficient, the commander of the blood has no strength and thus the movement of the blood becomes unsmooth. This easily results in stasis with static blood obstructing internally. This then prevents the blood from returning to its channels, and therefore, the qi and blood become even more vacuous. For this reason, the clinical manifestations of this condition are a mixture of vacuity and repletion.

The treatment of this condition largely utilizes qi-boosting medicinals, since when the qi becomes effulgent, the blood will be restrained and when qi is sufficient, stasis will automatically be transformed. In addition, when qi and blood are both effulgent and flourishing, the *chong* and *ren* will be regulated and harmonized. Within this formula, Codonopsis, Pseudostellaria, Astragalus, Atractylodes, Poria, and Licorice boost the qi and restrain the blood, supporting the righteous and securing the root. *Dang Gui*, Rehmannia, Cornus, and Dipsacus supplement and boost the liver and kidneys, nourish the blood and regulate the menses. Cyperus rectifies the qi and regulates the *chong*. *Shi Xiao San*, carbonized *Guan Zhong*, and powdered Pseudoginseng transform stasis and stop bleeding while at the same time insuring that there is no retention of stasis because of stopping bleeding. Thus, when these medicinals are used in combination, they have the functions of boosting the qi and nourishing the blood, transforming stasis and stopping bleeding and this is why this protocol gets good results.

Ectopic Pregnancy

"The Chinese Herbal Treatment of Ectopic Pregnancy" by Cui Hua-ming *et al.*, *Si Chuan Zhong Yi (Sichuan Traditional Chinese Medicine)*, #7, 1993, p. 43; BF

In this clinical audit, the authors report on the treatment of 10 cases of ectopic pregnancy seen from June 1990-March 1991. The women ranged in age from 23-35 years old. Their periods had ceased but there was irregular bleeding from the vagina and abdominal pain. Urine pregnancy tests were positive for 8 cases and negative for 2. The diagnosis of ectopic pregnancy was derived by physical examination.

The treatment method consisted of two formulas. Formula I: Radix Trichosanthis Kirlowii (_Tian Hua Fen_), 30g, Scolopendra Subspinipes (_Wu Gong_), 2 pieces, Radix Salviae Miltiorrhizae (_Dan Shen_), 15g, Rhizoma Sparganii (_San Leng_), Rhizoma Curcumae Zedoariae (_E Zhu_), Semen Pruni Persicae (_Tao Ren_), Radix Saussureae Seu Vladimiriae (_Mu Xiang_), Rhizoma Cyperi Rotundi (_Xiang Fu_), and Flos Carthami Tinctorii (_Hong Hua_), 10g @, processed Gummum Olibani (_Ru Xiang_) and Myrrha (_Mo Yao_), 8g @, Herba Leonuri Heterophylli (_Yi Mu Cao_), 20g, and raw Radix Glycyrrhizae (_Sheng Gan Cao_), 6g.

Formula II: Radix Salviae Miltiorrhizae (_Dan Shen_), 15g, Radix Rubrus Paeoniae Lactiflorae (_Chi Shao_), Rhizoma Ligustici Wallichii (_Chuan Xiong_), Rhizoma Corydalis Yanhusuo (_Yuan Hu_), and Cortex Cinnamomi (_Gui Pi_), 9g @, Rhizoma Sparganii (_San Leng_), Rhizoma Curcumae Zedoariae (_E Zhu_), Semen Pruni Persicae (_Tao Ren_), and Sclerotium Poriae Cocos (_Yun Ling_), 6g @. If there was qi vacuity, Radix Astragali Membranacei (_Huang Qi_), 9g, and processed Radix Rehmanniae (_Shu Di_), 15g, were added. If there was flooding and leaking (_i.e._, uterine bleeding), _Shi Xiao San_ (Loss of Smile Powder) was added. During administration of Formula I, when urine pregnancy tests turned negative or serological markers had lowered on 2 occasions, Formula I was stopped and Formula II was administered instead. Formula I kills the embryo, quickens the blood, and stops pain, while Formula II is for the purpose of quickening static blood, stopping pain, and opening the network vessels.

131

In this study, cure was defined as disappearance of the clinical manifestations as well as the physical manifestations revealed on examination. After administering formula I for 3 days, 3 cases' urine pregnancy text turned negative, with another five cases turning negative after 5 days administration. Nine cases were hospitalized for an average of 21 days for complete cure to be affected. One case was hospitalized for two months because of encysted blood accumulations on both sides of her abdomen which reabsorbed slowly.

"The Treatment of 15 Cases of Ectopic Pregnancy with *Yi Qi Huo Xue Tang* (Boost the Qi & Quicken the Blood Decoction)" by Ha Xiao-lian & Peng Hui-min, *Tian Jin Zhong Yi (Tianjin Traditional Chinese Medicine)*, #3, 1993, p. 12-3; BF

In this clinical audit, 15 cases of ectopic pregnancy were treated with *Yi Qi Huo Xue Tang*. Four of the women were between 24-26 years of age, 8 were between 27-30, and 3 were between 31-35 years old. In addition, 8 were primiparas, 6 had been pregnant twice, and 1 had been pregnant 3 times. Thirteen of the women had tubal pregnancies, 1 women had a uterine angle pregnancy, and 1 woman had an abdominal cavity pregnancy.

The formula used consisted of: Radix Angelicae Sinensis (*Dang Gui*), 9g, Radix Rubrus Paeoniae Lactiflorae (*Chi Shao Yao*), 9g, raw Pollen Typhae (*Sheng Pu Huang*), 9g, Gummum Olibani (*Ru Xiang*), 6g, mix-fried Myrrha (*Zhi Mo Yao*), Radix Linderae Strychnifoliae (*Wu Yao*), 9g, Rhizoma Cyperi Rotundi (*Xiang Fu*), 10g, Rhizoma Sparganii (*San Leng*) and Rhizoma Curcumae Zedoariae (*E Zhu*), 9g @, Radix Codonopsis Pilosulae (*Dang Shen*), 15g, Radix Salviae Miltiorrhizae (*Dan Shen*), 15g, and Radix Trichosanthis Kirlowii (*Tian Hua Fen*), 12g. These were decocted in 300 ml and administered 1 *ji* per day. the purpose of this formula was to boost the qi and nourish the blood, quicken the blood and transform stasis, and to rectify the qi and stop pain.

If abdominal pain was severe, Feces Trogopterori Seu Pteromi (*Ling Zhi*), 10g, was added and Lindera was increased to 15g. If hemorrhaging was excessive, Sparganum and Zedoaria were removed and Herba Leonuri Heterophylli (*Yi Mu Cao*), 15g, was added. If the appetite was poor, stir-fried Fructus Germinatus Hordei Vulgaris (*Chao Mai Ya*), 10g, and Endothelium Corneum Gigeriae Galli (*Nei Jin*), 6g, were added. And if there was constipation, Radix Et Rhizoma Rhei (*Chuan Jun*), 10g, or Folium Sennae (*Fan Xie Ye*), 3 g, were added.

Of the 15 cases so treated, all were completed cured except for 1 who was hemorrhaging greatly and received surgery. In their concluding discussion, the authors say that Red Peony, *Dang Gui*, Pollen Typhae, and Salvia quicken the blood and transform stasis, open the channels and stop pain. Frankincense, Myrrh, Sparganium, Zedoaria, Lindera, and Cyperus move the qi and break stasis, stop pain and disperse the conglomerations. Together, Codonopsis and Salvia supplement the qi and nourish the blood. The authors also say that ectopic pregnancy is usually a simultaneous vacuity and repletion condition, although repletion is dominant. If blood-quickening, stasis-transforming, and conglomeration-dispersing medicinals are used exclusively, the qi will follow the discharge of the blood. Therefore, in the treatment of this condition, it is essential to prevent the qi and blood from both becoming vacuous. The old Chinese doctor, Ha Li-tian, has pointed out that in this disease, "While treating by quickening the blood and transforming stasis, it is essential to use Fructus Germinatus Hordei Vulgaris, Fructus Crataegi (*Shan Zha*), Endothelium Corneum Gigeriae Galli, and other such medicinals to rectify the spleen and stomach, increase food and drink, and thus support the righteous while simultaneously transforming stasis and scattering nodulation."

"The Treatment of 21 Cases of Ectopic Pregnancy with Quickening the Blood & Transforming Stasis Method" by Jia Ying, *Jiang Su Zhong Yi (Jiangsu Traditional Chinese Medicine)*, #9, 1993, p.15-6; BF

The author begins this report by stating that traditionally this condition was discussed under lower abdominal depression of blood, concretions and conglomerations, falling fetus, etc. If, for some reason, surgery cannot be used to treat this condition, the methods of quickening the blood and transforming stasis may be resorted to. Of the 21 cases treated by these means by the author, 6 were between 23-30 years of age and 15 between 31-42. There were 16 cases of fallopian tube pregnancy, 4 cases of ovarian pregnancy, case of abdominal cavity pregnancy, and 1 cases of uterine cervix pregnancy. The author attributes this condition to a number of factors, such as lack of regulation of the *chong* and *ren* resulting in stasis and stagnation blocking and obstructing the *chong mai* and post-surgical obstruction and stagnation of the *bao mai*, all of which result in a blood stasis repletion pattern or blood stasis in the lower abdomen pattern. Based on this diagnosis, the authors says that the treatment principles are to quicken the blood and transform stasis, soften the hard and stop pain.

The formula employed is called *Huo Luo Xiao Ling Dan Jia Wei* (Quickening the Connecting Vessels Miraculously Effective Elixir with Added Flavors). It is comprised of: Radix Rubrus Paeoniae Lactiflorae (*Chi Shao*), Semen Pruni Persicae (*Tao Ren*), Gummum Olibani (*Ru Xiang*), Myrrha (*Mo Yao*), Rhizoma Sparganii (*San Leng*), and Rhizoma Curcumae Zedoariae (*E Zhu*).

If there was heat, Flos Lonicerae Japonicae (*Yin Hua*), Fructus Forsythiae Suspensae (*Lian Qiao*), Herba Cum Radice Taraxaci Mongolici (*Pu Gong Ying*), and Caulis Sargentodoxae (*Hong Teng*) were added. If there was cold, Fructus Evodiae Rutecarpae (*Wu Zhu*) and Ramulus Cinnamomi (*Gui Zhi*) were added. If there was bowel repletion (*i.e.*, constipation), Radix Et Rhizoma Rhei (*Da Huang*) and

Mirabilitum (*Mang Xiao*) were added. If there was abdominal pain, Pollen Typhae (*Pu Huang*), Feces Trogopterori Seu Pteromi (*Ling Zhi*), and Rhizoma Corydalis Yanhusuo (*Yan Hu*) were added. If there was discharge of copious blood, Radix Rubiae Cordifoliae (*Qian Cao*), Crinis Carbonisatus (*Xue Yu Tan*), and carbonized Fructus Crataegi (*Shan Zha Tan*) were added. If there was qi vacuity, Radix Astragali Membranacei (*Huang Qi*) and Radix Codonopsis Pilosulae (*Dang Shen*) were added. If the embryo was not dead, Radix Trichosanthis Kirlowii (*Tian Hua Fen*) or Scolopendra Subspinipes (*Wu Gong*) was added. If the absorption and assimilation of the bloody swelling was delayed, Flos Carthami Tinctorii (*Hong Hua*), Squama Manitis (*Chuan Shan Jia*), and Semen Vaccariae Segetalis (*Wang Bu Liu Xing*) were added. If there was nausea and vomiting, Pericarpium Citri Reticulatae (*Chen Pi*) and Rhizoma Pinelliae Ternatae (*Ban Xia*) were added. And if intake (*i.e.*, appetite) was below normal, Massa Medica Fermentata (*Shen Qu*) and Endothelium Corneum Gigeriae Galli (*Ji Nei Jin*) were added.

In this study, complete cure was defined as disappearance of the signs and symptoms of this condition, disappearance of lower abdominal pain, cessation of blood flowing from the vaginal tract, the menses returning to normal, and serum pregnancy indicators either disappearing or being reduced by 2/3. Based on these criteria, the author reports that all 21 cases were completely cured. The author also says that, in the treatment of this disease, it is typically not appropriate to use heavy doses of blood-stopping medicinals since these might impede the assimilation and reabsorption of static blood.

"The Treatment of 40 Cases of Unruptured Fallopian Tube Pregnancy by Quickening the Blood & Transforming Stasis" by Wu Lian-zhen, *Zhe Jiang Zhong Yi Za Zhi (Zhejiang Journal of Traditional Chinese Medicine)*, #7, 1993, p. 304-5; BF

Dr. Wu begins this report on the treatment of ectopic pregnancy by saying that the methods of quickening the blood and transforming stasis were used in order to promote miscarriage. Thirty women in this study were between 23-28 years of age and 10 were over 30 with the oldest being 50 years old. In 3 cases, their menstruation had ceased less than 35 days previously. In 28 cases, their menses had ceased between 35-40 days before, in 7 cases 41-45 days before, and in 2 cases more than 46 days before. Pregnancy was confirmed by cessation of menstruation, urine test, serum tests, lower abdominal distention and pain, and pelvic examinations. Based on these criteria, all the women in this group were diagnosed as suffering from tubal pregnancy.

The author states that tubal pregnancy may be due to the three causes of 1) the seven orientations (*i.e.*, emotions), 2) the six wanton (evils), and 3) external injury. These injure and damage the *chong* and *ren* so that they do not flow smoothly and uninhibited. The *chong* and *ren* become obstructed and stagnant and accumulating blood becomes conglomerations and concretions. Therefore, appropriate treatment should quicken the blood, transform stasis, and disperse conglomeration, course and rectify the *chong* and *ren* and regulate the menstruation.

The medicinals commonly used for these purposes were: Radix Salviae Miltiorrhizae (*Dan Shen*), Radix Rubrus Paeoniae Lactiflorae (*Chi Shao*), Rhizoma Sparganii (*San Leng*), and Rhizoma Curcumae Zedoariae (*E Zhu*), 15g @, and Semen Pruni Persicae (*Tao Ren*), Gummum Olibani (*Ru Xiang*), and Myrrha (*Mo Yao*), 10g @.

If the tongue was pale with a white coating and the pulse was deep and slow, Cortex Cinnamomi (_Rou Gui_), 5g, and Radix Praeparatus Aconiti Carmichaeli (_Shu Fu Pian_), 10g, were added. If the tongue was red with a yellow coating and the pulse was wiry and rapid, Flos Lonicerae Japonicae (_Yin Hua_) and Fructus Forsythiae Suspensae (_Lian Qiao_), 15g @, were added. If the abdomen was distended, Fructus Citri Seu Ponciri (_Zhi Ke_) and Cortex Magnoliae Officinalis (_Hou Pu_), 5g @, were added, and if there was constipation, raw Radix Et Rhizoma Rhei (_Sheng Da Huang_), 10g, was added.

After administration of from 10-30 _ji_ of the above medicinals, 36 cases were cured, meaning their urine pregnancy tests turned negative, their serum pregnancy markers disappeared, and their menses returned to normal. Four cases experienced no result. In other words, their urine pregnancy tests remained positive, their serum pregnancy markers remained, the lumps in their abdomen increased in size, or their tubes ruptured. Among the cases which experienced no result, 3 were treated surgically when their urine and serum tests did not change and the lumps in their abdomen grew larger. The other case experienced rupture of their tube and fever, at which time they were also treated surgically.

Excessive Amniotic Fluid

"The Treatment of Acute Excessive Amniotic Fluid Using _Ling Gui Zhu Gan Tang Jia Wei_ (Poria, Cinnamon, Atractylodes, & Licorice Decoction with Added Flavors" by Chu Guan-jin & Yue Jia-yi, _Shang Hai Zhong Yi Yao Za Zhi (The Shanghai Journal of Traditional Chinese Medicine & Medicinals)_, #11, 1993, p. 22-3; BF

The authors report that they have treated 32 cases of acute excessive amniotic fluid with _Ling Gui Zhu Gan Tang Jia Wei_ between 1980-

1989. This is called *yang shui guo duo* in the modern TCM literature and is essentially the same as *zi mian*, child fullness, in the traditional literature. The ages of these 32 cases ranged from 24-35. Twenty-four were between 24-30 and 8 were between 31-35, with most of these being between 28-30. Twenty-eight were primiparas and the rest were multiparas. The onset of this condition typically manifests between the 4-6th months of pregnancy, with 24 of these women developing this condition in the 5th month. Symptoms of this condition include abnormal enlargement of the abdomen, fullness and oppression of the chest and diaphragm, forced, urgent breathing, and dyspnea counter-flow which will not be quieted and which, in severe cases, prohibits lying flat. Twenty-five of the women in this study also had edematous swelling of their lower extremities and external genitalia, while 7 cases generalized edema. These women's tongue were pale and fat with a white, slimy coating, and their pulses were deep, slippery, and forceful.

The formula consisted of: Ramulus Cinnamomi (*Gui Zhi*), 5g, Sclerotium Poriae Cocos (*Fu Ling*), 12g, Rhizoma Atractylodis Macrocephalae (*Bai Zhu*), 12g, Radix Angelicae Sinensis (*Dang Gui*), 10g, Radix Albus Paeoniae Lactiflorae (*Bai Shao*), 10g, raw Cortex Rhizomatis Zingiberis (*Sheng Jiang Pi*), 5g, Pericarpium Arecae Catechu (*Da Fu Pi*), 10g, Cortex Radicis Mori (*Sang Bai Pi*), 10g, Radix Glycyrrhizae (*Gan Cao*), 5g, and carp, 1 tailpart (*i.e.*, approximately 1/2 kilo with viscera removed). These were added to a suitable amount of water and decocted into soup. The herbs were removed and the remaining liquid was divided into 2 drinks per day. If there was severe abdominal distention, Rhizoma Alismatis (*Ze Xie*), 10g, and Semen Plantaginis (*Che Qian Zi*, wrapped during decoction), 10g, were added. If the spirit was exhausted and there was lack of strength with qi vacuity, Radix Astragali Membranacei (*Huang Qi*), 15g, was added. If there was kidney vacuity with low back ache, Semen Cuscutae (*Tu Si Zi*) and Ramus Loranthi Seu Visci (*Ji Sheng*), 12g @, were added. If the face was whitish and there was blood vacuity, Gelatinum Corii Asini (*E Jiao*), 10g, and Radix Polygoni

138

Multiflori (*Shou Wu*), 10g, were added. And if there was severe urgent dyspneic breathing, Semen Pruni Armeniacae (*Xing Ren*), 10g, was added.

After 7 days of treatment, 22 cases were cured, meaning that their symptoms disappeared. After 15 days, another 7 cases were cured. However, 3 cases experienced no result after 15 days of treatment.

Vaginal Itch

"Semen Cnidii Monnieri Powder for 204 Cases of Trichomoniasis (&) Mycotic Pudendal Itching" by Rao Gui-zhen, *Shang Hai Zhong Yi Yao Za Zhi (The Shanghai Journal of Traditional Chinese Medicine & Medicinals)*, #9, 1992, p. 12; BF

This research report describes both the treatment and its success rate. The ages of the women in the study ranged from 17-53 years old. Seventy-three cases were between 17-25 years of age; 98 cases between 26-45; and 33 cases between 46-53. The duration of their disease went from 3 days to more than 2 years. One hundred thirteen cases had gone on for 3 days to 3 months; 80 cases for more than 3 months to 1 year, and 11 cases from more than 1 year to more than 2 years.

The formula used was *She Chuang Zi San* (Cnidium Powder): Semen Cnidii Monnieri (*She Chuang Zi*), 30g, Radix Sophorae Flavescentis (*Ku Shen*), 30g, Radix Stemonae (*Bai Bu*), 30g, Fructus Zanthoxyli Bungeani (*Hua Jiao*), 15g, and Alum (*Ming Fan*), 20g.

This formula was created at the Shanghai College of Traditional Chinese Medicine. If itching was severe, 30g of Rhizoma Smilacis Glabrae (*Tu Fu Ling*) was added. If there were excessive vaginal secretions, 30g of Cortex Phellodendri (*Huang Bai*) and 20g of Radix Ledebouriellae Sesloidis (*Fang Feng*) were added. These medicinals were placed in water and boiled for 15 minutes. The women then fumigated their genitalia with the steam rising off this decoction for approximately 20 minutes each time, 2 times per day. After fumigation, they also washed their genitalia with this decoction. One *ji* of herbs was used per day and 10 days' treatment equalled 1 course of therapy.

Of the 204 cases, 179 were completely cured or 87.75%. Of these, 143 were diagnosed as suffering from trichomoniasis vaginalis and the other 36 suffered from yeast infections. Another 22 cases markedly improved or 10.78%. Of these, 18 had trichomoniasis and 4 yeast infections. Three cases experienced no result or 1.47%. Two of these women were diagnosed as suffering from trichomoniasis and 1 from mycosis. Of the cases that were completely cured, 93 cases were cured in between 5-12 days, 81 cases in 13-21 days, 25 cases in 22-28 days, and 2 cases in 29-42 days. The total amelioration rate for this treatment protocol was 98.53%.

Cervical Cancer

"The Pattern Discrimination Treatment of Stone Conglomeration (*i.e.*, Cervical Cancer)" by Wang Yu-jing, *Bei Jing Zhong Yi (Beijing Traditional Chinese Medicine)*, #6, 1993, p. 59-60; BF

The author begins this article by saying that stone conglomeration (*shi jia*) is the same as cervical cancer (*zi gong jing ai*). This is a malignant tumor disease which occurs in women. It mostly arises in adult women, women who have had numerous pregnancies, or women who have married too early. The majority of cases occur in women between 40-50 years of age with some cases occuring between 50-60.

It is rarely seen in women before 20 years of age.

In discussing the causes and mechanisms of this disease, the author states that many cases of this disease are due to menstrual or postpartum damage and injury of the *chong* and *ren* with external invasion of damp toxins gathering and obstructing the *bao luo*. It may also be due to liver qi depression and binding. In this case, coursing and discharge lose their regularity, resulting in qi stagnation, blood stasis. Then static blood accumulates and binds. It is also possible for spleen vacuity to generate dampness. Dampness may then accumulate and transform into heat. Over a long period, these become toxins and damp toxins pour downward. Further, due to bodily vacuity weakness, the *bao mai* may experience deficiency detriment. This may be associated with either yang vacuity or yin deficiency conditions. Thus, long-term worry, anxiety, depression, and anger may result in internal damage by the seven emotions. This, in turn, may become involved with the six wanton evils and toxins. In addition, loss of control either during gestation, postpartum, or over bedroom affairs may damage the liver and cause detriment to the spleen, eventually affecting the kidneys. The *chong* and *ren* may thus lose regularity and qi and blood may become chaotic. Damp toxins may accumulate internally, and thus this disease may arise.

Treatment Based on Pattern Discrimination

1. Liver depression, spleen dampness pattern

Signs & symptoms: Increasingly copious abnormal vaginal discharge which is yellow in color and like pus or red and white simultaneously and which may occasionally have a bad odor, lower abdominal aching and pain, a depressed, oppressed essence spirit, chest and lateral costal distention and fullness, torpid intake, a low fever, heart vexation, dry mouth, a red or purple tongue with a yellow, slimy coating, and a slippery, rapid, or wiry or choppy pulse

Treatment principles: Soothe the liver and fortify the spleen, eliminate dampness and resolve toxins

Rx: Radix Bupleuri (*Chai Hu*), Rhizoma Smilacis Glabrae (*Tu Fu Ling*), Flos Lonicerae Japonicae (*Yin Hua*), Sclerotium Polypori Umbellati (*Zhu Ling*), Rhizoma Alismatis (*Ze Xie*), Rhizoma Imperatae Cylindricae (*Bai Mao Gen*), Sichuan Rhizoma Dioscoreae Hypoglaucae (*Chuan Bi Xie*), Semen Plantiginis (*Che Qian Zi*), Apex Radicis Angelicae Sinensis (*Gui Wei*), Radix Rubrus Paeoniae Lactiflorae (*Chi Shao*), Radix Dioscoreae Oppositae (*Shan Yao*), and Herba Oldenlandiae (*Bai Hua She She Cao*)

2. Qi & yin dual vacuity pattern

Signs & symptoms: Increasingly copious abnormal vaginal discharge, typically bleeding from the vaginal meatus, possible flooding or leaking downward, low back soreness and weak lower limbs, four limbs fear of chill, spirit fatigued, torpid intake, possible vexatious heat in the five hearts, dizziness, ringing in the ears, a pale, fat tongue with a thin white coating and peeled patches, and a fine, rapid, forceless pulse

Treatment principles: Nourish yin and boost the qi, clear and resolve toxic evils

Rx: Radix Glehniae Littoralis (*Bei Sha Shen*), raw Radix Astragali Membranacei (*Sheng Huang Qi*), Rhizoma Smilacis Glabrae (*Tu Fu Ling*), Radix Codonopsis Pilosulae (*Dang Shen*), Rhizoma Imperatae Cylindricae (*Bai Mao Gen*), Fructus Ligustri Lucidi (*Nu Zhen Zi*), Ramus Loranthi Seu Visci (*Sang Ji Sheng*), Nidus Vespae (*Feng Fang*), Semen Cuscutae (*Tu Si Zi*), Herba Ecliptae Prostratae (*Han Lian Cao*), Radix Dioscoreae Oppositae (*Shan Yao*) and Periostracum Serpentis (*She Tui*)

For external use, apply *Hei Jiang Dan* (Black Downbearing Elixir) 1 time per day if the lesion has already ulcerated and ruptured.

Case history: Female, 45 years old, married, worker. In January, 1984, the patient had been diagnosed as suffering from cervical cancer at another hospital where she was immediately admitted and treated surgically. Three months after surgery, she came to the Beijing Traditional Chinese Medicine Hospital for a diagnosis. She was extremely uncomfortable about her condition. However, she only had a comparatively excessive white vaginal discharge. Otherwise, her appetite was normal and her urination and defecation were regular and harmonious. Gynecologic examination revealed cervical erosion and an area which was slightly red. Her tongue coating was white and slimy and her pulse was wiry and slippery. Therefore, her condition was categorized as spleen dampness and liver depression, damp heat pouring downward.

Treatment consisted of fortifying the spleen and soothing the liver, clearing heat and disinhibiting dampness. The formula was composed of: Rhizoma Smilacis Glabrae (*Tu Fu Ling*), 30g, Tuber Curcumae (*Yu Jin*), 10g, Radix Bupleuri (*Chai Hu*), 10g, Hangzhou Radix Albus Paeoniae Lactiflorae (*Hang Bai Shao*), 10g, Herba Polygoni Avicularis (*Bian Xu*), 10g, Herba Dianthi (*Qu Mai*), 10g, Flos Lonicerae Japonicae (*Jin Yin Hua*), 20g, Herba Cum Radice Taraxaci Mongolici (*Pu Gong*), 30g, Talcum (*Hua Shi*), 20g, and raw Radix Glycyrrhizae (*Sheng Gan Cao*), 10g. Externally, *Hei Jiang Dan* was applied to the cervical erosion 1 time per day. After 3 whole months of administration of the above formula, the disease's condition was certainly stabilized.

Menopausal Syndrome

"Suggestions for Treating Menopausal Syndrome with *Er Xian Tang* (Two Immortals Decoction)" by Zheng Yu-lan, *Shan Dong Zhong Yi Za Zhi (The Shandong Journal of Traditional Chinese Medicine)*, #6, 1992, p. 25-6; BF

In this article, Zheng Yu-lan gives several modifications of *Er Xian Tang* for the treatment of menopausal syndrome. According to Zheng, this formula balances and supplements kidney yin and yang, drains liver fire, and balances the *chong* and *ren*. Treatment was based on pattern discrimination

1. Loss of balance between yin and yang with yin vacuity predominating

The signs and symptoms of this pattern include red cheeks of the face, sweating, easy weeping with grief, easy anger, heart vexation, sleep not tranquil, hands, feet, and heart hot, a pale, red tongue with a red tip and thin, white coating, and a wiry, fine, rapid or deep, fine, wiry, rapid pulse. In this case, the therapeutic principles are to enrich kidney yin, drain liver fire, and balance the *chong* and *ren* assisted by warming kidney yang. For this purpose, use *Er Xian Tang Jia Wei* (Two Immortals Decoction with Added Flavor): Rhizoma Curculiginis Orchoidis (*Xian Mao*), 6g, Herba Epimedii (*Yin Yang Huo*), 6g, Radix Morindae Officinalis (*Ba Ji Tian*), 6g, Radix Angelicae Sinensis (*Dang Gui*), 15g, Rhizoma Anemarrhenae (*Zhi Mu*), 12-15g, Cortex Phellodendri (*Huang Bai*), 9-15g, and Radix Albus Paeoniae Lactiflorae (*Bai Shao*), 12-15g.

2. Loss of balance between yin and yang with yang vacuity predominating

The signs and symptoms include periodic redness of the cheeks,

144

sweating, vexation and agitation, fear of cold, typically also fear of chill, or loose stools, a pale red tongue whose body is comparatively fat and tender with a thin, white coating, and a deep, fine, forceless or slightly rapid pulse. In this case, the therapeutic principles are to warm kidney yang, balance the *chong* and *ren* assisted by enriching kidney yin and draining liver fire. The formula suggested consists of: Rhizoma Curculiginis Orchoidis (*Xian Mao*), 15g, Herba Epimedii (*Yin Yang Huo*), 15g, Radix Morindae Officinalis (*Ba Ji Tian*), 15g, Radix Angelicae Sinensis (*Dang Gui*), 12g, Rhizoma Anemarrhenae (*Zhi Mu*), 6g, and Cortex Phellodendri (*Huang Bai*), 6-9g.

3. Loss of balance between yin and yang with blood vacuity predominating

The signs and symptoms include episodes of flushing of the cheeks of the face, sweating, heart vexation, heart palpitations, dizziness, lack of strength, insomnia, a pale red tongue or a red tongue tip with a thin, white coating, and a deep, fine, forceless pulse. The therapeutic principles in this case are to balance yin and yang, supplement the *chong* and *ren*, boost the qi, nourish the blood, enrich yin, and clear heat. The formula suggested is *Er Xian Tang Jia Wei* (Two Immortals Decoction with Added Flavors): Rhizoma Curculiginis (*Xian Mao*), 6g, Herba Epimedii (*Yin Yang Huo*), 6g, Radix Morindae Officinalis (*Ba Ji Tian*), 6g, Radix Angelicae Sinensis (*Dang Gui*), 15g, Rhizoma Anemarrhenae (*Zhi Mu*), 12-15g, Cortex Phellodendri (*Huang Bai*), 9-15g, Radix Albus Paeoniae Lactiflorae (*Bai Shao*), 12-15g, Caulis Polygoni Multiflori (*Ye Jiao Teng*), 30g, and Fructus Zizyphi Jujubae (*Da Zao*), 7 pieces.

4. If heart palpitations, dizziness, and lack of strength are prominent, increase Radix Angelicae Sinensis (*Dang Gui*) to 20g and add Radix Astragali Membranacei (*Huang Qi*), 30g. If the stools are parched and dry, add Semen Biotae Orientalis (*Bai Zi Ren*), 30g.

"The Treatment of Female Climacteric Edema with *Xiao Yao San Jia Wei* (Rambling Powder with Added Flavors)" by Ren Qing-wen & Chun Zhu-ying, *Si Chuan Zhong Yi (Sichuan Traditional Chinese Medicine)*, #6, 1993, p. 40; BF

This clinical audit discusses the treatment of 30 cases of menopausal edema using *Xiao Yao San Jia Wei*. The women were between 45-54 years old. The longest course of disease was 6 years and the shortest was half a year. The edema was worse in the facial area upon arising in the morning and worse in the lower extremities after noon. This was accompanied by loss of sleep, heart palpitations, tenseness, agitation, and easy anger, heart vexation, dizziness, and erratic periods coming early or late. Plus the amount of the menses was excessive.

The formula used to treat these women consisted of: Radix Bupleuri (*Chai Hu*), Radix Angelicae Sinensis (*Dang Gui*), Radix Rubrus Et Albus Paeoniae Lactiflorae (*Chi Bai Shao*), Semen Plantaginis (*Che Qian Zi*), Sclerotium Poriae Cocos (*Fu Ling*), Rhizoma Atractylodis Macrocephalae (*Bai Zhu*), Pericarpium Viridis Citri Reticulatae (*Qing Pi*), Rhizoma Cyperi Rotundi (*Xiang Fu*), Fructus Citri Seu Ponciri (*Zhi Ke*), Herba Ephedrae (*Ma Huang*), and Caulis Akebiae Mutong (*Mu Tong*).

If there was abdominal pain before the period with a lot of blood clots, Radix Salviae Miltiorrhizae (*Dan Shen*) and Semen Pruni Persicae (*Tao Ren*) were added. If there was loss of sleep and excessive dreams, heart vexation and heart palpitations, Radix Polygalae Tcnuifoliae (*Yuan Zhi*), prepared Semen Zizyphi Spinosae (*Zhi Zao Ren*), and Sclerotium Pararadicis Sclerotii Poriae Cocos (*Fu Shen*) were added. If there was dizziness and headache, raw Os Draconis (*Long Gu*), Fructus Tribuli Terrestris (*Bai Ji Li*), Flos Chrysanthemi Morifolii (*Ju Hua*), and Ramulus Uncariae Seu Uncis (*Gou Teng*) were added. If there was low back and knee weakness, Rhizoma Curculiginis Orchoidis (*Xian Mao*), Herba Epimedii (*Xian*

Ling Pi), Radix Morindae (*Ba Ji Tian*), and Cortex Eucommiae Ulmoidis (*Du Zhong*) were added.

Complete cure consisted of the water swelling disappearing with no return after half a year and obvious reduction in the other symptoms. Marked improvement consisted of the water swelling disappearing but recurring within half a year. When this was administered again, again the edema went away. In addition, the other symptoms were reduced. Based on these criteria, 18 women were cured, 10 were markedly improved, and only 2 experienced no result. Thus the total amelioration rate was 93%. Treatment lasted from as short as 15 days to as long as 2 whole months.

Yang He Tang

"Recent Developments in the Clinical Use of *Yang He Tang* (Yang Harmonizing Decoction) in Gynecology" by Zhang Yi-qing & Lu Ming-hui, *Bei Jing Zhong Yi (Beijing Traditional Chinese Medicine)*, #6, 1993, p. 55; BF

In this essay, the authors survey recent developments in the use of *Yang He Tang* in gynecology as reported in various articles published in a number of Chinese TCM journals from 1984-1990. This formula is from the Qing dynasty book, *Wai Ke Quan Sheng Ji (A Complete Collection of [Patterns & Treatments] in External Medicine)*, by Wang Wei-de. It consists of seven flavors: prepared Radix Rehmanniae (*Shu Di*), Semen Sinapis Albae (*Bai Jie Zi*), Gelatinum Cornu Cervi (*Lu Jiao Jiao*), Cortex Cinnamomi (*Rou Gui*), blast-fried Rhizoma Zingiberis (*Pao Jiang*), Herba Ephedrae (*Ma Huang*), and raw Radix Glycyrrhizae (*Sheng Gan Cao*). These ingredients have the ability to warm yang and supplement the blood, scatter cold and open stagnation. Originally this formula was created to treat yin *ju* (*i.e.*, deep-rooted ulcer) conditions in external medicine. However, this formula

147

has been used to treat a variety of gynecological diseases with good results, and, over the past 10 years, a number of articles have been published on its use in gynecology.

Ovarian cysts

Master Li (as reported in *Zhong Yi Za Zhi [The Journal of Traditional Chinese Medicine]*, #11, 1989, p. 40) used this formula with Semen Pruni Persicae (*Tao Ren*), Herba Sargassii (*Hai Zao*), and Rhizoma Curcumae Zedoariae (*E Zhu*) added to treat 26 cases of ovarian cysts. In this study, 23 cases were cured, meaning their cysts completely disappeared, 2 cases got some result, meaning that their cysts became smaller and their symptoms either disappeared or diminished, and 1 case got no result. Of those who were cured, the smallest number of *ji* was 5 and the largest was 36.

Master Hu (as reported in *Jiang Su Zhong Yi Za Zhi [The Jiangsu Journal of Traditional Chinese Medicine]*, #9, 1987, p. 22) also used this formula to treat a single case of ovarian cyst by adding Radix Albus Paeoniae Lactiflorae (*Bai Shao*), Radix Angelicae Sinensis (*Dang Gui*), and Sclerotium Poriae Cocos (*Fu Ling*) and changing Cortex Cinnamomi to Ramulus Cinnamomi (*Gui Zhi*). The cyst was 14 x 14 x 12cm in size. After administering approximately 57 *ji*, the cyst completely disappeared.

Stein-Leventhal Syndrome

Master Shen (as reported in *Zhe Jiang Zhong Yi Za Zhi [The Zhejiang Journal of Traditional Chinese Medicine]*, #8, 1986, p. 373) used this formula to successfully treat one case of amenorrhea and Stein-Leventhal Syndrome by adding Rhizoma Curculiginis Orchoidis (*Xian Mao*), Herba Epimedii (*Xian Ling Pi*), Radix Angelicae Sinensis (*Dang Gui*), and Radix Morindae Officinalis (*Ba Ji Tian*). Previously, the woman had lost a lot of blood postpartum and this had led to amenorrhea, uterine atrophy, and Stein-Leventhal Syndrome. After administering 10 _ji_ of these medicinals, the period came on. On follow-up a half year later, the woman was pregnant and eventually gave birth to a boy.

Endometriosis

Master Chen (as reported in _Si Chuan Zhong Yi [Sichuan Traditional Chinese Medicine]_, #3, 1988, p. 19) first administered 10 _ji_ of a number blood-quickening, stasis-transforming medicinals in a case of endometriosis. However, these were without effect. Therefore, he used this formula with Radix Angelicae Sinensis (_Dang Gui_), Feces Trogopterori Seu Pteromi (_Wu Ling Zhi_), Rhizoma Cyperi Rotundi (_Xiang Fu_), etc. Before each period, he administered 3 _ji_, and after three months, the menstruation was normal and the symptoms had disappeared. On follow-up 2 years later, there had been no recurrence.

Infertility

Master Liu (as reported in _Bei Jing Zhong Yi [Beijing Traditional Chinese Medicine]_, #5, 1986, p. 43) added Radix Astragali Membranacei (_Huang Qi_), Rhizoma Atractylodis Macrocephalae (_Bai Zhu_), Sclerotium Poriae Cocos (_Fu Ling_), Semen Nelumbinis Nuciferae (_Lian Zi_), Semen Cuscutae (_Tu Si Zi_), and Radix Morindae Officinalis (_Ba Ji Tian_) to this formula to treat a single case of infertility which had persisted for 5 years. After administering this formula for 4 months, the woman conceived.

Breast Lump

Master Sun (writing in _Bei Jing Zhong Yi [Beijing Traditional Chinese Medicine]_, #4, 1985, p. 20) added Bulbus Fritillariae Thunbergii (_Zhe Bei Mu_), Fructus Trichosanthis Kirlowii (_Gua Lou Ke_), Rhizoma Cyperi Rotundi (_Xiang Fu_), and Radix Rubrus Paeoniae Lactiflorae

(*Chi Shao*) and subtracted the blast-fried Ginger to treat a single case of breast lump. After administering 20 *ji* of these medicinals, the lump disappeared. On follow-up 1 year later, there had been no recurrence.

Dysmenorrhea

Master Yang (as reported in *Bei Jing Zhong Yi [Beijing Traditional Chinese Medicine]*, #10, 1984, p. 45) used this formula to treat dysmenorrhea with good results by adding Rhizoma Atractylodis Macrocephalae (*Bai Zhu*), Feces Trogopterori Seu Pteromi (*Wu Ling Zhi*), Rhizoma Cyperi Rotundi (*Xiang Fu*), and Fructus Foeniculi Vulgaris (*Xiao Hui Xiang*).

Amenorrhea

Master Cui (as reported in *Hu Nan Zhong Yi Za Zhi [The Hunan Journal of Traditional Chinese Medicine]*, #2, 1987, p. 39) used this formula with good results to treat blood vacuity, yang debility amenorrhea by adding Folium Artemesiae Argyii (*Ai Ye*), Radix Codonopsis Pilosulae (*Dang Shen*), Rhizoma Ligustici Wallichii (*Chuan Xiong*), Rhizoma Cyperi Rotundi (*Xiang Fu*), and Radix Achyranthis Bidentatae (*Niu Xi*).

Vaginal Discharge & Uterine Bleeding

Another Master Shen (as reported in *Bei Jing Zhong Yi [Beijing Traditional Chinese Medicine]*, #4, 1987, p. 52) treated a woman with this formula who had excessive white vaginal discharge and flooding (*i.e.*, heavy uterine bleeding). In this case, the practitioner added Cornu Degelatinum Cervi (*Lu Jiao Shuang*), Semen Trigonellae Foenigraeci (*Hu Lu Ba*), and Os Sepiae Seu Sepiellae (*Wu Zei Gu*). In this case, 3 *ji* achieved a good effect.

Post-abortion Painful *Bi*

Master Shi (as reported in *Jiang Su Zhong Yi Za Zhi [The Jiangsu Journal of Traditional Chinese Medicine]*, #2, 1990, p. 14) used this formula to treat 57 cases of post-abortion painful *bi*. In this study, Dr. Shi used heavy doses of Rehmannia and added Radix Albus Paeoniae Lactiflorae (*Bai Shao*), 45-60g. Forty-three cases were cured, 11 got good results, and 3 experienced no improvement for a total amelioration rate of 94.7%.

In addition, reports on the successful use of this formula for excessive menstruation (*Xin Zhong Yi [New Traditional Chinese Medicine]*, #11, 1988, p. 59), flooding and leaking (*Fu Jian Zhong Yi Yao [Fujian Traditional Chinese Medicine & Medicinals]*, #2, 1986, p. 59), and pelvic inflammatory disease (*Zhong Yi Za Zhi [The Journal of Traditional Chinese Medicine]*, #10, 1984, p. 45) have also been published.

Nan Ke
Urology & Male Sexual Dysfunction ___

Impotence

"A Clinical Discussion of 130 Cases of Damp Heat Impotence Treated by *Liu Miao Tang* (Six Wonders Decoction)" by Zhao Shou-yun & Xu Xiang-zhi, *Hu Bei Zhong Yi Za Zhi (The Hubei Journal of Traditional Chinese Medicine)*, #5, 1993, p. 25; BF

This is a report on a clinical audit conducted between 1986-1992 on 130 cases of damp heat impotence. Of the 130 men, 31 cases were between 20-30 years of age, 42 between 31-40, and 57 were over 40 years of age. Thirty-two cases had suffered from this condition for less than 1 year, 49 from 1-2 years, 27 from 2-3 years, 14 from 3-4 years, and 8 cases had suffered for 5 years or more. In addition, 78 cases had accompanying lower abdominal lurking pain and 32 had scrotal damp itch (*i.e.,* eczema). Most cases also had reddish yellow or cloudy, turbid urine. Their tongue coating was white and thick and their pulse was sodden and rapid.

The formula for their treatment was composed of: Rhizoma Atractylodis (*Cang Zhu*), Radix Stephaniae Tetrandrae (*Fang Ji*), Cortex Phellodendri (*Huang Bai*), and Radix Achyranthis Bidentatae (*Niu Xi*), 12g @, Semen Coicis Lachryma-jobi (*Yi Yi Ren*), 30g, and Fructus Chaenomelis Lagenariae (*Mu Gua*), 15g. These are to be decocted in water and taken, each day 2 doses.

If there is simultaneous kidney yin vacuity as manifest by low back and knee soreness and pain, vertigo and dizziness, and ringing in the ears, combine (the above) with *Liu Wei Di Huang Tang* (Six Flavors Rehmannia Decoction) with additions and subtractions. If there is simultaneous spleen vacuity as manifest by an emaciated physical form, weak limbs, and lack of strength, add Rhizoma Atractylodis Macrocephalae (*Bai Zhu*) and Radix Dioscoreae Oppositae (*Shan Yao*) to strengthen the spleen and boost the qi. And if there are simultaneously the appearance of dribbling, dripping, astringent, and painful urination, add Talcum (*Hua Shi*) and Folium Bambusae (*Zhu Ye*) to disinhibit urination and open strangury.

Of the 130 cases, 78 were completed cured as evidenced by their ability to achieve and maintain and erection, have normal sexual intercourse, and the disappearance of accompanying symptoms. Forty-two experienced a fair result, meaning that they could achieve and erection, the erection was comparatively firm, or, even though their erection was not firm, they were able to ejaculate. Ten cases experienced no result. This meant that they experienced no change in their symptoms after treatment as compared to before and were still not able to have sexual relations.

In their concluding discussion, the authors say that though impotence is many times treated in clinical practice as kidney vacuity, injury and damage of the spleen and stomach may cause accumulation and stagnation giving rise to dampness. In that case, long(-standing) depression transforms in heat, and damp heat pours downward (or to the lower [burner]), there causing vertical slackness in the ancestral sinew. This then results in yang affairs not (being able) to rise up. Within *Liu Miao Tang, Er Miao San* (Three Wonders Pills) clears heat and dries dampness, Coix clears heat and disinhibits dampness, Stephania increases strength and eliminates dampness, and Achyranthis and Chaenomeles free the connecting vessels and soothe the sinews. Thus dampness is dispelled and heat cleared, the ancestral sinew is returned to normal, and this leads to the automatic cure of impotence.

"The Treatment of 93 Cases of Impotence with *Shu Gan Wen Shen Ning Xin Tang* (Course the Liver, Warm the Kidneys, & Tranquilize the Heart Decoction)" by Xu Chao, *He Nan Zhong Yi (Henan Traditional Chinese Medicine)*, #9, 1993, p. 231; BF

This clinical audit reports on the treatment of 93 cases of impotence treated with *Shu Gan Wen Shen Ding Xin Tang* which the authors composed themselves. Of the 93 cases, the youngest was 24 and the oldest was 48, with the average age being 36.3 years old. The shortest disease duration was 20 days and the longest was 3 years, with the average duration of disease being 6.5 months. According to the authors, 20 cases were due to prolonged masturbation. Nine cases were due to excessive sexual activity (1 or more times per day). Thirteen cases were due to excessive worry and anxiety. Fifteen cases were due to fright. Thirteen cases were due to drinking iced water after sex. Eighteen cases were due to psychological depression. And 5 cases were due to addiction to alcohol.

The formula consisted of: Radix Bupleuri (*Chun Chai Hu*), 9g, Fructus Meliae Toosendan (*Chuan Lian Zi*), 12g, stir-fried Radix Albus Paeoniae Lactiflorae (*Chao Bai Shao*), 15g, Radix Angelicae Sinensis (*Quan Dang Gui*), 12g, Fructus Cnidii Monnieri (*She Chuang Zi*), 12g, processed Rhizoma Curculiginis Orchoidis (*Zhi Xian Mao*), 10g, Herba Epimedii (*Xian Ling Pi*), 12g, Nidus Vespae (*Lu Feng Fang*), 9g, mix-fried Radix Polygalae Tenuifoliae (*Zhi Yuan Zhi*), 10g, Semen Zizyphi Spinosae (*Suan Zao Ren*), 12g, Flos Albizziae Julibrissinis (*He Huan Hua*), 12g, and mix-fried Radix Glycyrrhizae (*Zhi Gan Cao*), 6g.

If there were signs of vacuity cold, Radix Praeparatus Aconiti Carmichaeli (*Fu Pian*) and Cortex Cinnamomi (*Rou Gui*) were added. If there were apparent signs of blood stasis, Radix Cyathulae (*Chuan Niu Xi*), Semen Pruni Persicae (*Tao Ren*), and Fructus Liquidambaris

155

Taiwaniae (*Lu Lu Tong*) were added. If there was yin vacuity and internal heat, Rhizoma Anemarrhenae (*Zhi Mu*), Cortex Phellodendri (*Huang Bai*), Cortex Radicis Moutan (*Dan Pi*), and raw Radix Rehmanniae (*Sheng Di*) were added. If there was liver/gallbladder damp heat, Radix Gentianae Scabrae (*Long Dan Cao*), Semen Plantaginis (*Che Qian Zi*), and Rhizoma Alismatis (*Ze Xie*) were added. If there was qi vacuity, Radix Codonopsis Pilosulae (*Dang Shen*), Rhizoma Atractylodis Macrocephalae (*Bai Zhu*), and Radix Astragali Membranacei (*Huang Qi*) were added. If there was blood vacuity, Fructus Lycii Chinensis (*Gou Qi Zi*) and prepared Radix Rehmanniae (*Shu Di*) were added. If there was more severe liver depression, Pericarpium Viridis Citri Reticulatae (*Qing Pi*) and Rhizoma Cyperi Rotundi (*Xiang Fu*) were added. If kidney vacuity was not obvious, Curculiginis and Epimedium were subtracted. If simultaneously there were spermatorrhea and premature ejaculation, Fructus Alpiniae Oxyphyllae (*Yi Zhi Ren*) and Fructus Corni Officinalis (*Shan Zhu Yu*) were added.

The above formula was decocted in water and administered internally, 1 *ji* per day, with 15 days equalling 1 course of treatment. At the same time, patients received psychological counselling. During treatment, administration of any other Western or Chinese medicines was stopped. Patients were advised against drinking alcohol and were forbidden to have sex.

Cure was defined as ability to achieve and sustain and erection and to have successful sexual relations with no relapse within 1 year. Improvement was defined as ability to achieve an erection but not necessarily be able to sustain it, with sometimes successful sex and sometime unsuccessful sex or recurrence of the condition within 1 year. No result meant that there was no obvious improvement in erectile potency after 3 whole courses of treatment and intercourse was still difficult or unsuccessful. Based on these criteria, 66 cases or 70.9% were cured, 21 case or 22.7% were improved, and 6 cases or 6.4% experienced no result. Thus the combined amelioration rate was

93.6%. Among those who received a result from this treatment, the shortest duration of treatment was 10 days and the longest was 60 days, with the average being 28.5 days.

According to the authors in their concluding discussion, impotence is not due to anything other than the two causes of vacuity and repletion. Vacuity is divided into kidney vacuity and heart/spleen dual vacuity types. Repletion types consist of liver depression, damp heat, yin cold, and blood stasis. There are also mixed vacuity/repletion types as well. Among the *zang fu* involved in the disease mechanisms at work in this disease, the heart, liver, and kidneys are the three main viscera, and clinically all three are most commonly involved together. Therefore, within *Shu Gan Wen Shen Ding Xin Tang*, Bupleurum, Melia, *Dang Gui*, and White Peony course the liver and resolve depression, nourish the blood and relax the liver. Curculiginis, Epimedium, Cnidium, and Nidus Vespae warm the kidneys, fortify yang, and raise up the atonic (*i.e.*, flaccid). Polygala, Ziziphus Spinosa, and Flos Albizziae Julibrissinis calm the heart and resolve depression, quiet the spirit and stabilize the orientation (*i.e.*, the emotions). Licorice harmonizes the center and regulates and harmonizes the other medicinals. Thus, these medicinals when used together treat the heart, liver, and kidneys at the same time. They have the ability to course the liver and calm the heart, warm the kidney, and raise up the atonic.

Sperm Anomalies

"A Brief Discussion of 35 Cases of Asthenospermia Treated by *Qiang Jing Jian* (Strengthen the Essence Decoction)" by Sun Jie-ping, *Jiang Su Zhong Yi (Jiangsu Traditional Chinese Medicine)*, #11, 1993, p. 14; BF

In this clinical audit, 35 men were treated Chinese herbal medicine for infertility due to asthenospermia. Twenty-three men were 30 years old or younger. Twelve men were between the ages of 31-40. Five cases had not been able to successfully fertilize their partner in a half year. Eighteen had not been able to fertilize their partner in from 1-2 years. And twelve had not been able to fertilize their partner in more than 2 years of trying. Among this group there were anomalies in amount of seminal fluid, sperm count and motility, and lower than normal pH.

The formula used, *Qiang Jing Jian*, was comprised of: Prepared Radix Rehmanniae (*Shu Di Huang*), Radix Dioscoreae Oppositae (*Huai Shan Yao*), Fructus Corni Officinalis (*Shan Zhu Yu*), Radix Angelicae Sinensis (*Quan Dang Gui*), and Fructus Lycii Chinensis (*Gou Ji Zi*), 12g @, Placenta Hominis (*Zi He Che*), mix-fried Bombyx Batryticatus (*Zhi Jiang Can*), and dried Lumbricus (*Gan Di Long*), 15g @, Herba Cistanchis (*Rou Cong Rong*) and Cornu Cervi (*Lu Jiao Pian*), 10g @. If there was simultaneous yin vacuity with effulgent fire, Tuber Ophiopogonis Japonicae (*Mai Dong*) and Plastrum Testudinis (*Gui Ban*), 10g @, were added. If there was damp heat in the lower burner, Cortex Phellodendri (*Huang Bai*) and Semen Plantaginis (*Che Qian Zi*), 10g @, were added. If there was stasis and obstruction of the seminal pathway, Rhizoma Ligustici Wallichii (*Chuan Xiong*) and Semen Vaccariae Segetalis (*Wang Bu Liu Xing Zi*), 10g @, were added. And if there was kidney yang deficiency and vacuity, Herba Epimedii (*Xian Ling Pi*) and Radix Morindae (*Ba Ji Tian*), 10g @, were added. One *ji* was given per day with 2 months equalling 1 course of treatment. During the course of treatment, alcohol was prohibited, and patients were instructed that it would be better to restrict normal sexual activity.

After treatment with *Qiang Jing Jian,* of the 35 cases with less than class II sperm motility, 27 had between class II-III motility. Of the 25 cases who had had a motility rate below 50%, 18 cases had a motility rate in excess of 60%. In addition, in a significant number of cases, pH rose to more normal levels. Interestingly, the author did not include either a discussion of the TCM mechanisms associated with seminal abnormalities nor the TCM rationale for the basic formula used. Although, from an analysis of its ingredients, it is clear that its aim is to primarily supplement the kidneys and fulfill the essence.

Prostatitis

"The Treatment of Chronic Prostatitis with *Jia Jian Huo Xue Xiao Ling Dan* (Modified Quicken the Blood Miraculously Effective Elixir) as a Retention Enema" by Luo Yirong, *Bei Jing Zhong Yi Za Zhi (The Beijing Journal of Traditional Chinese Medicine)*, #2, 1993, p. 32-3; BF

Huo Xue Xiao Ling Dan is originally found in the *Yi Xue Zhong Zhong Can Xi Lu (Records of Heart-felt Experiences in the Study of Medicine with Reference to the West)*. The author has used it as a retention enema for the treatment of chronic prostatitis in 84 patients since 1986. The ages of the patients ranged from 19-59 years old. Sixty-two or 73.8% were between 19-39, and 23 were unmarried. The course of disease had lasted from 8 months to 12 years, with 45 cases or 53.6% having had this problem for 1 year, 37 cases or 44% from 1-10 years, and 2 cases for 12 years. Seventy-nine or 94% of these patients had used other treatments without success. Their symptoms included 1) various types of sexual dysfunction: impotence, spermatorrhea, premature ejaculation, and sterility in 7 cases, 2) various types and locations of pain: coccygeal pain, perineal pain, perianal pain, lower abdominal pain, penile and testicular pain, and sore pain on the inner side of the thigh, 3) various urinary disturbances: urinary pain, frequent urination, urinary urgency, a burning hot feeling, hematuria, etc., 4) generalized symptoms: loss of sleep, fear of cold, fever, lack of strength, dizziness, tinnitus, and emaciation, and 5) rectal examination revealed enlargement or hardening.

The formula consisted of: Gummum Olibani (*Ru Xiang*), 30g, Myrrha (*Mo Yao*), 30g, Radix Angelicae Sinensis (*Dang Gui*), 30g, Radix

Dipsaci (*Xu Duan*), 30g, and Caulis Sargentodoxae (*Da Huo Xue*), 50g. These were decocted in water 2 times, resulting in 200ml of fluid. This was allowed to cool until the temperature was about 41°C. The patient was instructed to lay down on his back and draw up their knees. This decoction was then administered as a retention enema once every other day. Ten such treatments equalled 1 course of treatment. During this treatment the patient was prohibited to drink alcohol or engage in any sexual activity.

Forty-eight men or 57.2% experienced marked improvement from this treatment, including the complete disappearance of their symptoms. Twenty-eight men or 33.3% experienced satisfactory results, meaning that their symptoms either disappeared or were reduced. And 8 men or 9.5% experienced no result from this treatment. Thus the combined amelioration rate was 90.5%.

"The Treatment of 136 Cases of Chronic Prostatitis" by Qiao Bao-jun, Qiao Zhen-gang, & Wang Li-jun, *Hu Nan Zhong Yi Za Zhi (The Hunan Journal of Traditional Chinese Medicine)*, #1, 1993, p. 12-4; BF

In this research report, the authors discuss their treatment of 136 cases of chronic prostatitis. The men in this study ranged in age from 23-51 years of age. There were 22 cases among men 40-50 years old, 49 cases among those 30-39 years old, and 54 cases among those 20-29 years old. The average age was 34.7 years old. The duration of disease went from as long as 31 years to as short as half a year. The average course of disease was 4.3 years. The perineal area was hard, distended, and uncomfortable in 112 cases or 82.4%. Ninety-two cases (67.6%) experienced a white, turbid discharge either before or after urination. Fifty-eight cases (42.6%) experienced low back soreness, aching, and pain. Seventy-two cases (52.9%) complained of diminished sexual function. And 13 married men (9.6%) suffered from sterility.

The formula used was *Qian Lie Shu Fang* (Prostate Coursing Formula): Radix Salviae Miltiorrhizae (*Dan Shen*), 15g, Cortex Radicis Moutan (*Dan Pi*), 9g, Cortex Phellodendri (*Huang Bai*), Radix Rubrus Paeoniae Lactilforae (*Chi Shao*), Squama Manitis Pentadactylis (*Chuan Shan Jia*), and Herba Lycopi Lucidi (*Ze Lan*), 10g @, Rhizoma Alismatis (*Ze Xie*) and Rhizoma Dioscoreae Hypoglaucae (*Chuan Bi Xie*), 15g @, Pericarpium Viridis Citri Reticulatae (*Qing Pi*) and Semen Vaccariae Segetalis (*Wang Bu Liu Xing*), 9g @, Herba Cum Radice Taraxaci Mongolici (*Pu Gong Ying*), 15g, Semen Pruni Persicae (*Tao Ren*), 7g, Radix Linderae Strychnifoliae (*Wu Yao*), 7g, and Herba Patriniae Heterophyllae (*Bai Jiang Cao*), 30g.

These ingredients were decocted in water and drunk each morning and evening. The dregs were decocted in water and used as a sitz bath every evening. One month equalled 1 course of therapy. In addition, patients were instructed to gently massage their perineum once per day. They were counselled to avoid stimulating foods and alcohol, and sexual activity was also restricted.

Thirty-one cases (22.8%) experienced complete cure; 43 cases (31.6%), marked improvement; 51 cases (37.5%), some improvement; and 11 cases (8.1%), no improvement. Thus the total amelioration rate was 91.8%. However, the best percentages of cure and improvement occurred in those whose disease had lasted from 3-10 years. In addition, the highest percentage of those registering either cure or improvement did so after 4-6 courses, *i.e.*, months, of treatment. Further, men between the ages of 30-39 responded better statistically than those either older or younger.

According to Qiao *et al.*, this protocol is primarily designed to treat damp heat in the liver channel with qi stagnation, stasis, and obstruction. It clears heat and disinhibits dampness, rectifies the qi and transforms stasis. Because chronic prostatitis is a replete branch or

161

biao condition existing with a root vacuity, after the symptoms are eliminated, one should supplement the kidneys and consolidate the root.

Prostatic Hypertrophy

The Treatment of 25 Cases of Prostatic Hypertrophy with *Qian Lie Xiao Chong Ji* (Prostate Dispersing Soluble Granules" by Zhang Shen-lan, *Jiang Su Zhong Yi (Jiangsu Traditional Chinese Medicine)*, #2, 1993, p. 16; BF

This clinical audit describes the treatment of 25 cases of prostatic hypertrophy with *Qian Lie Xiao Chong Ji*, a patent medicine made as a desiccated extract. The principles upon which this preparation was formulated were to course and rectify the qi and blood, soften the hard and scatter nodulation, disperse accumulations and open and disinhibit.

Qian Lei Xiao Chong Ji consists of: Radix Astragali Membranacei (*Huang Qi*), Cortex Cinnamomi (*Rou Gui*), mix-fried Radix Et Rhizoma Rhei (*Zhi Da Huang*), Apex Radicis Angelicae Sinensis (*Gui Wei*), Semen Pruni Persicae (*Tao Ren*), Squama Manitis Pentadactylis (*Shan Jia*), Semen Vaccariae Segetalis (*Wang Bu Liu Xing*), Fructificatio Polypori Mylittae (*Lei Wan*), Spica Prunellae Vulgaris (*Xia Gu Cao*), Herba Sargassii (*Hai Zao*), and Rhizoma Smilacis Glabrae (*Tu Fu Ling*).

The proportions of the above medicinals in this preparation were 3 : 0.9 : 1 : 1.5 : 1 : 1.5 : 1 : 1 : 3 : 1.5 : 3. One packet was taken each time, 2 times per day. This preparation was marked effective in all cases in this study. In his explanation of the formula, Dr. Zhang explains that prostatic hypertrophy is a common disease among older men. He quotes the classic, saying, "At 8 (times) 8 the kidney qi becomes deficient." Kidney deficiency leads to lower burner vacuity cold and thus to qi stagnation and blood stasis. Phlegm turbidity binds with this and accumulation results in the formation of lumps which obstruct and hinder the water passageway. The bladder loses its power and there is difficulty urinating. Therefore, the root is vacuous and the branch is replete and this protocol seeks to support the root while at the same time as draining repletion.

Er Ke
Pediatrics _____

Hyperactivity

"A Discussion of Pediatric Hyperactivity" by Du Yu-qi, *Shan Dong Zhong Yi Za Zhi (The Shandong Journal of Traditional Chinese Medicine)*, #6, 1992, p. 55; BF

In a case history discussion, Du Yu-qi discusses pediatric hyperactivity (*xiao er guo dong zheng*). Dr. Du attributes this in the case under discussion to insufficiency of prenatal kidney water or essence which then fails to nourish liver wood. This 6 year old child's signs and symptoms included a weak body, sparse hair which tended to be fine and yellowish, emotional anxiety and agitation, sweating excessively at night, occasional dry stools, a normal tongue, and a fine pulse. Based on this, Dr. Du prescribed *Liu Wei Di Huang Tang Jia Wei* (Six Flavors Rehmanniae Decoction with Added Flavors): Radix Rehmanniae (*Sheng Di*), 9g, prepared Radix Rehmanniae (*Shu Di*), 9g, Cortex Radicis Moutan (*Dan Pi*), 9g, Radix Albus Paeoniae Lactiflorae (*Bai Shao*), 12g, Sclerotium Poriae Cocos (*Fu Ling*), 9g, Rhizoma Alismatis (*Ze Xie*), 9g, Radix Achyranthis Bidentatae (*Niu Xi*), 9g, Fructus Corni Officinalis (*Shan Zhu Yu*), 9g, Concha Ostreae (*Sheng Mu Li*), 20g, and Os Draconis (*Sheng Long Gu*), 20g. These were decocted in water and taken in divided doses, 1 *ji* or formula, *i.e.*, packet, per day. After 25 *ji*, his condition was improved. He was switched to *Liu Wei Di Huang Wan* (Six Flavors Rehmannia Pills) and continued on these for 1 full month more. At that point, the disease was cured.

Bronchitis

"40 Cases Utilizing Shang Shi Zhi Tong Gao (Damage by Dampness, Stop Pain Plasters) as an Adjunctive Therapy in the Treatment of Capillary Bronchitis" by Chen Jian-cong, Zhong Guo Zhong Xi Yi Za Zhi (Chinese Journal of Integrated Chinese-Western Medicine), #2, 1992, p. 123; BF

In this study, *Shang Shi Zhi Tong Gao* (Damage by Dampness, Stop Pain Plaster) was used as an adjunctive therapy in the treatment of 40 cases of pediatric bronchitis. Plasters were applied bilaterally to *Fei Shu* (Bl 13) for a duration of 12 hours. Three applications constituted 1 course of treatment. The youngest patients were less than 6 months old and the oldest were more than 2 years old. The duration of the illness ranged from 1-7 days with the average being 2.05 days. Thirty-six of the cases were of common severity; 3 cases were severe; and 1 was extremely severe.

(In these cases,) the primary therapy of choice was antibiotics. However, the authors maintain that the plasters were particularly effective in resolving symptoms of asthmatic breathing and obstructed airway stemming from bronchitis. (*Shang Shi Zhi Tong Gao* is readily available in the U.S.)

"The Treatment of 840 Cases of Pediatric Cough With An Fei Gao (Quiet the Lungs Plasters) Applied to Acupoints" by Wang Qi-ming & Zhang Xin-jian, Zhe Jiang Zhong Yi Za Zhi (The Zhejiang Journal of Traditional Chinese Medicine), #1, 1993, p. 34; BF

This large clinical audit describes the treatment of 840 cases of pediatric cough by applying _An Fei Gao_ (Quiet the Lungs Plasters) over acupoints. This study lasted over a period of 2 years.

An Fei Gao consists of: Fructus Gleditschiae Chinensis (_Zao Jiao_), 150g, Cordyceps Sinensis (_Dong Chong Xia Cao_), 6g, Radix Glycyrrhizae (_Gan Cao_), 6g, raw Rhizoma Pinelliae Ternatae (_Sheng Ban Xia_), 15g, raw Rhizoma Arisaematis (_Sheng Nan Xing_), 15g, Sclerotium Poriae Cocos (_Fu Ling_), 30g, Semen Lepidii (_Ting Li Zi_), 30g, Pericarpium Citri Erythrocarpae (_Hua Ju Hong_), 20g, raw Radix Aconiti (_Sheng Chuan Wu_), 10g, Pulvis Margaritae (_Zhen Zhu Fen_), 3g, Pulvis Ligni Aquilariae Agallochae (_Chen Xiang Wei_), 3g, Borneol (_Bing Pian_), 9g, and Gecko (_Ge Jie_), 1 pair

The above medicinals were fried in roasted sesame oil (_Xiang You_), except for the Margarita, Borneol, and Pulvis Ligni Aquilariae Agallochae. The dregs were removed and the resulting liquid was strained. The decoction was heated again and Minium (_Huang Dan_) was added until a paste is formed. The resulting mixture was poured into cold water and left immersed for 15 days. The water was changed twice per day to clear fire toxins. The paste was cut into small pieces and steamed until soft. The powdered medicinals reserved above were then added, mixing them in thoroughly. This paste was stored for later use. When used, a 1 _cun_ in diameter flat pieces of this plaster was placed over _Fei Shu_ (Bl 13) bilaterally and _Shan Zhong_ (CV 17). These plasters were left in place for 3 days.

Of the 840 cases, 501 were males and 339 were females. One hundred seventy-two ranged in age from 5 months to 1 year; 376 from 2-3 years; and 292 from 4-8 years of age. Further, 532 had been diagnosed as suffering from upper respiratory infection and 308 from bronchitis. Treatment lasted from 3-6 days. After that length of time, 588 were obviously improved, 240 were somewhat improved, and only 12 registered no improvement. Thus the total amelioration rate was 98.02%.

Diarrhea

"The Treatment of 96 Cases of Pediatric Diarrhea Using *Huo Xiang Zheng Qi San* (Agastaches Righteous Qi Powder)" by Gao Hong-lan, *Shan Dong Zhong Yi Xue Yuan Xue Bao (Journal of the Shandong College of traditional Chinese Medicine)*, Vol. 17, #1, 1993, p. 39; CC

This clinical audit discusses the treatment of 96 cases of pediatric diarrhea with *Huo Xiang Zheng Qi San*. The children's symptoms included fever, nausea, and diarrhea with 5 or more bowel movements per day. The ages of the patients ranged from 6 months to 3 years old. A single *ji* of *Huo Xiang Zheng Qi San* was decocted in 80-100 ml of water and divided into 3-5 doses per day.

The formula consists of: Herba Agastachis Seu Pogostemmi (*Huo Xiang*), 5-10g, Pericarpium Arecae Catechu (*Da Fu Pi*), 5-10g, Folium Perillae Frutescentis (*Zi Su*), 4-6g, Rhizoma Atractylodis Macrocephalae (*Bai Zhu*), 5-15g, Radix Angelicae (*Bai Zhi*), 5-10g, Sclerotium Poriae Cocos (*Fu Ling*), 5-15g, Cortex Magnoliae Officinalis (*Hou Po*), 5-10g, Rhizoma Pinelliae Ternatae (*Ban Xia*), 4-6g, Pericarpium Citri Reticulatae (*Chen Pi*), 5-10g, Radix Platycodi Grandiflori (*Jie Geng*), 5-10g, and Radix Glycyrrhizae (*Gan Cao*), 3-5g.

If there was watery stools, Sclerotium Polypori Umbellati (*Zhu Ling*), 5-10g, was added. If there was no fever, Angelica, Platycodon, and Perilla were deleted. If there was no vomiting, Pinellia, Angelica, Perilla, and Platycodon were deleted.

If the fever abated, vomiting ceased, and the stools normalized with 4 small bowel movements per day in infants up to 6 months and 2 bowel movements per day in children 6 months to 3 years, this was considered a cure. Diarrhea was arrested in 12-48 hours in 8 cases and in 48-72 hours in 24 cases.

Case history: Female, 18 months old. The patient had had a fever for 2 days with projectile vomiting, diarrhea, and 7 bowel movements per day. She received some (unspecified) treatment and her temperature decreased. However, her vomiting and diarrhea persisted. She was in good spirits, her mouth was dry, and she was agitated. Her temperature was 37.4°C. Her tongue was pale with a slimy, white coating. Her digital vein was pale red at the qi gate. Her stools were yellow, the color of cornsilk. She was given 3 _ji_ of _Huo Xiang Zheng Qi San_ and all her symptoms disappeared.

Huo Xiang Zheng Qi San is for the treatment of externally contracted wind cold and internal damage due to damp turbidity. This external contraction of wind cold checks the spreading of protective yang, resulting in aversion to cold and fever. Internal injury due to damp turbidity impairs spleen function, producing gastric fullness, oppression, borborygmus, and abdominal pain. It also causes the qi to counterflow, causing nausea and vomiting. The clear yang sinks, resulting in diarrhea. Because children have weak digestions and tend to be damp, when they get sick, they typically have a fever, vomiting, and diarrhea.

Tourette's Syndrome

"The Treatment of 52 Cases of Pediatric Tourette's Syndrome Based on the Lungs" by Xu Zhu-qian, _Zhong Yi Za Zhi (Journal of Traditional Chinese Medicine)_, #11, 1993, p. 678-9; BF

This clinical audit reports on the treatment of 52 cases of pediatric Tourette's Syndrome. In Chinese, this is called _chou dong yi hui yu zeng he zheng_. This literally translates as twitching & foul language syndrome. The study was conducted from February 1991 to February 1992. Of the 52 cases, 41 were boys and 11 were girls. They ranged in age from a minimum of 4 years old to a maximum of 15, with the median age being 9. The course of disease had lasted from a minimum of 3 months to a maximum of 12 years, with a median duration of 2 years 8 months.

The treatment consisted of decocting Flos Magnoliae (*Xin Yi*), 10g, Fructus Xanthii (*Cang Er Zi*), 10g, Radix Scrophulariae Ningpoensis (*Yuan Shen*), 10g, Radix Isatidis Seu Baphicacanthi (*Ban Lang Gen*), 10g, Radix Sophorae Subprostratae (*Shan Dou Gen*), 5g, Rhizoma Pinelliae Ternatae (*Ban Xia*), 3g, Ramulus Uncariae Seu Uncis (*Gou Teng*), 10g, etc. The herbs were removed leaving approximately 100ml of fluid. This was divided into 4 doses per day and administered orally. Twenty-eight days equalled 1 course of treatment.

After 1 course of treatment, if the condition had returned to normal, this was defined as complete cure. If there was obvious reduction in twitching of more than 3/4, this was defined as marked improvement. If there was more than 1/2 reduction, this was defined as some improvement. And if there was no obvious improvement, this was defined as no result. Based on these criteria, 28 cases or 53.8% of the children in this study were cured. Seventeen cases or 32.7% experienced marked improvement. Five cases or 9.6% experienced some improvement. And only 2 cases or 3.8% experienced no result.

Case history: Girl, 9 years old. The child experienced uncontrollable twitching of the eyelids, corners of the mouth, neck, abdomen, and four limbs. There was a repetitive, odd sound in her throat, her nose was blocked and not open, and her appetite was a little reduced. Her two excretions (*i.e.*, urination and defecation) were regular. Her facial color was somber white and without lustre. Her tongue was slightly red with a slimy, slightly yellow coating. Her pulse was slippery and had strength. Electroencephalogram (EEG) and CAT scan were without apparent abnormality. She was diagnosed as suffering from Tourette's syndrome which was categorized as wind phlegm attached to the lungs. Having been prolonged and not dispelled from the upper clear portals, this caused the squeezed brows, blinking eyes, stuffed nose, and shrugging shoulders. Further, this had poured into the channels and connecting vessels resulting in twitching movements of the body and limbs.

Treatment was to dispel wind and open the portals, clear the lungs and sweep phlegm. The medicinals used consisted of: Flos Magnoliae (*Xin Yi*), 10g, Fructus Xanthii (*Cang Er Zi*), 10g, Radix Scrophulariae Ningpoensis (*Yuan Shen*), 10g, Radix Isatidis Seu Baphicacanthi (*Ban Lang Gen*), 10g, Radix Sophorae Subprostratae (*Shan Dou Gen*), 5g, Rhizoma Pinelliae Ternatae (*Ban Xia*), 3g, Ramulus Uncariae Seu Uncis (*Gou Teng*), 10g, Buthus Martensis (*Quan Xie*), 3g, Scolopendra Subspinipes (*Wu Gong*), 1 piece. After taking 10 *ji* of the above formula, the strange sound in the throat, squeezing of the brows, blinking of the eyes, etc. were brought under control and the twitching movements of the body and limbs were markedly reduced. However, the patient still had the stuffed nose and reduced appetite. Therefore, the above formula was continued with various additions and subtractions. After another 13 *ji*, the child's body no longer twitched. Her appetite was still reduced and her facial color was a lusterless, faded yellow. Her tongue was pale with a thin, white coating, and her pulse was fine and slippery.

At this point, the beating of wind and phlegm had more or less been levelled, but there was still lung spleen qi vacuity and the presence of dampness. Therefore, treatment to fortify the spleen and transform phlegm, supplement earth and generate metal was required to secure the treatment results. The formula used was *Liu Jun Zi Tang Jia Wei* (Six Gentlemen Decoction with Added Flavors): Radix Codonopsis Pilosulae (*Dang Shen*), 10g, Sclerotium Poriae Cocos (*Fu Ling*), 10g, stir-fried Rhizoma Atractylodis Macrocephalae (*Chao Bai Zhu*), 10g, stir-fried Radix Albus Paeoniae Lactiflorae (*Chao Bai Shao*), 10g, mix-fried Radix Glycyrrhizae (*Zhi Gan Cao*), 5g, Pericarpium Citri Reticulatae (*Chen Pi*), 5g, Rhizoma Pinelliae Ternatae (*Ban Xia*), 5g,

Buthus Martensis (*Quan Xie*), 3g, Ramulus Uncariae Seu Uncis (*Gou Teng*), 10g, Endothelium Corneum Gigeriae Galli (*Ji Nei Jin*), 10g, and parched Three Immortals (*Jiao San Xian*), 10g @. After 7 *ji* of this, the appetite was normal and there was no recurrence of the twitching.

However, there was heart vexation, heat in the hands, feet, and heart (or heat in the center of the hands and feet), a slightly red tongue with a slimy, slightly yellow coating, and a slippery pulse. This was again due to the lung and spleen qi. In this case, the power of movement and transformation was still not sufficient. Although appetite had returned to normal, food was accumulating and giving rise to internal heat. This then manifest as heart vexation and heat in the hands, feet, and heart. Once again it was necessary to strengthen the spleen and supplement the lungs, supplement earth and engender metal, but to also disperse food and transform phlegm. Thus, the above formula without the Scorpion and with 10g of Fructus Forsythiae Suspensae (*Lian Qiao*) added was given, after which everything was cured.

According to the author's discussion, most cases of Tourette's Syndrome are provoked by invasion of external evils resulting in beating of wind and phlegm. This is based on the saying, "Stubborn phlegm strange conditions are mostly due to phlegm making mischief." Wind's nature governs movement and twitching, and, if wind phlegm evils remain for a long time and are not removed, they harass the clear portal above, causing squeezing of the brows and blinking of the eyes. They raid the portal of the nose above, causing stuffy nose and shrugging. They congest the throat, causing itchy throat, repetitive strange noises, and unstoppable cursing. When they pour into the channels and connecting vessels, they result in endless twitching movement of the body and limbs. This disease is rooted in the lungs, and if lung disease continues for a long time, it will eventually reach the spleen. This is the child stealing the mother's qi. In that case, there will be dual lung/spleen vacuity. Therefore, treatment should first be directed at the lungs, dispelling wind and eliminating phlegm.

When wind and phlegm are removed, then lung/spleen qi vacuity images will be outstanding. Thus, after the primary symptoms of this condition have been eradicated, treatment should supplement the mother and boost the child by the methods of fortifying the spleen and boosting the lungs. When the defensive exterior is strong, it will be difficult for external evils to invade and there will be no further recurrence of this disease!

Pi Fu Ke
Dermatology _____

Anal Itch

"The Treatment of 62 Cases of Perianal Eczematous Itching with Self-composed Formulas" by Zhao Chun-lei & Lin Bo, *Ji Lin Zhong Yi Yao (Jilin Traditional Chinese Medicine & Medicinals)*, #4, 1993, p. 26; BF

The authors treated 62 cases of perianal eczematous itching with a combination of orally administered *Zhi Yang Fang* (Stop Itching Formula) and externally applied *Xun Xi Fang* (Fumigation & Wash Formula). Both these formulas were designed by the authors themselves. Of the 62 cases, 38 were men and 24 were women. They ranged in age from a low of 12 years to a high of 65 years old, with 41 between 30-45. Twenty-nine were workers, 18 were peasants, 11 were unemployed, and 4 were students. In 14 cases, their course of disease had lasted less than half a year. In 33 cases, it had lasted from 1-3 years, in 8 cases 4-6 years, in 5 cases 7-10 years, and in 2 cases more than 10 years. The shortest disease course was 3 months and the longest was 14 years.

The internal stop itching formula consisted of: Radix Rehmanniae (*Sheng Di*), 20g, Cortex Phellodendri (*Huang Bai*), 20g, Pericarpium Citri Reticulatae (*Chen Pi*), 20g, Cortex Radicis Dictamni (*Bai Xian Pi*), 20g, Semen Cnidii Monnieri (*She Chuang Zi*), 20g, Rhizoma Alismatis (*Ze Xie*), 15g, and Rhizoma Smilacis Glabrae (*Tu Fu Ling*), 15g. These were decocted in water and administered, 1 *ji* per day divided into 2 doses. If damp heat was more serious, Radix Sophorae Flavescentis (*Ku Shen*), 20g, and Semen Coicis Lachryma-jobi (*Yi Yi*

Ren), 20g, were added to this formula. If perianal itching was severe, Fructus Kochiae Scopariae (*Di Fu Zi*), 15g, was added. If there was blood vacuity giving rise to wind, *Si Wu Tang* (Four Materials Decoction) without Rhizoma Ligustici Wallichii (*Chuan Xiong*) was combined with this formula plus Herba Seu Flos Schizonepetae Tenuifoliae (*Jing Jie*), 15g, and Periostracum Cicadae (*Chan Tui*), 10g.

The external fumigation and wash formula consisted of: Radix Sophorae Flavescentis (*Ku Shen*), 50g, Semen Cnidii Monnieri (*She Chuang Zi*), 30g, Cortex Radicis Dictamni (*Bai Xian Pi*), 30g, Cortex Phellodendri (*Huang Bai*), 30g, Radix Ledebouriellae Sesloidis (*Fang Feng*), 20g, Folium Artemisiae Argyii (*Ai Ye*), 15g, Herba Seu Flos Schizonepetae Tenuifoliae (*Jing Jie*), 15g, and Borneol (*Bing Pian*), 5g. A suitable amount of water was added and the medicinals were decocted. Then the herbs were removed from the liquid. The affected part was fumigated for approximately 20 minutes and then, when the temperature was appropriate, the affected area was washed for about 2 minutes. This was done 2-3 times per day.

Complete cure consisted of the disappearance of the clinical condition after 15 days of treatment with no recurrence on follow-up in 1 year. Good improvement was defined as obvious diminishment of the clinical condition after 15 days of treatment. And no improvement was defined as no change in the clinical condition after 15 days. Based on these criteria, 54 cases were completely cured, 7 experienced good results, and only one case experienced no result. Thus the combined amelioration rate was 98.5%

Herpes Zoster

"46 Cases of Belt-like Herpes (*i.e.*, Herpes Zoster) Treated by *Jie Du Huan Ji Tang* (Resolve Toxins & Relax Tension Decoction)" by Bai Jun-feng & Tang Xing-shun, *Yun Nan*

Zhong Yi Za Zhi (The Yunnan Journal of Traditional Chinese Medicine), #5, 1993, p. 8; BF

In this clinical audit conducted in 1992, 46 cases of herpes zoster were treated by *Jie Du Huan Ji Tang*. Of the 46, 27 were men and 19 were women. Their ages ranged from 9-63 years old. Three cases had herpes lesions on their face, 2 on their neck, 32 on their torso, 3 on their upper extremities, 5 on their lumbosacral area, and 1 on their lower extremities. The composition of the formula used was based on the principles of clearing heat and resolving toxins, relaxing tension and stopping pain. The formula was composed of: Rhizoma Dryopteridis Seu Blechni (*Guan Zhong*), Fructus Chaenomeles Lagenariae (*Mu Gua*), raw Radix Albus Paeoniae Lactiflorae (*Sheng Bai Shao*), and raw Radix Glycyrrhizae (*Sheng Gan Cao*). Within this formula, *Guan Zhong* and Chaenomeles clear heat, disinhibit dampness, and resolve toxins, thus treating the cause of the condition. While Peony and Licorice relax tension, stop pain, and resolve toxins, thus treating the fruit (of the cause).

If heat was more serious, Flos Lonicerae Japonicae (*Yin Hua*) and Fructus Forsythiae Suspensae (*Lian Qiao*) were added to clear heat and resolve toxins. If dampness was more serious, Semen Coicis Lachryma-jobi (*Yi Yi Ren*) and Rhizoma Smilacis Glabrae (*Tu Fu Ling*) were added to disinhibit dampness and resolve toxins. If pain was more severe, Radix Clematidis Chinensis (*Wei Ling Xian*) and Rhizoma Corydalis Yanhusuo (*Yuan Hu*) were added to free the channels and stop pain. If there was accompanying stomach and intestinal problems, *Ping Wei San* (Level the Stomach Powder) was added to dry dampness and harmonize the stomach. And if there was pain and soreness as the lesions were dispersed and retreated, Gummum Olibani (*Ru Xiang*) and Myrrha (*Mo Yao*) were added to quicken the blood and transform stasis, move stagnation and stop pain.

177

Cure was defined as dispersal and retreat of the skin lesions and disappearance of (herpetic) neuralgia. Based on these criteria, all 46 cases were cured by this treatment. Treatment lasted between 2-9 days within which this extremely harmful condition responded.

"New Clinical Uses of *Da Chai Hu Tang* (Major Bupleurum Decoction)" by Yang Su-lan & Zhu Ye-ci, *He Nan Zhong Yi (Henan Traditional Chinese Medicine)*, #9, 1993, p. 212; BF

In this essay, the authors discuss a number of new clinical applications of *Da Chai Hu Tang*. This discussion includes a case history of herpes zoster. The patient was a 47 year old male who presented with fear of cold, fever, and red herpetic lesions on his left lateral costal region which were itchy and painful. In addition, he had a bitter taste in his mouth and dry throat, red urine, constipation, a thick, slimy tongue coating, and floating, wiry pulse. He was prescribed: Radix Bupleuri (*Chai Hu*), 9g, Radix Ledebouriellae Sesloidis (*Fang Feng*), 6g, Fructus Gardeniae Jasminoidis (*Zhi Zi*), 15g, Radix Scutellariae Baicalensis (*Huang Qin*), 12g, Fructus Immaturus Citri Seu Ponciri (*Zhi Shi*), 6g, Radix Et Rhizoma Rhei (*Da Huang*, added after), 12g, Radix Albus Paeoniae Lactiflorae (*Bai Shao*), 12g, and Rhizoma Coptidis Chinensis (*Huang Lian*), 10g. After 2 *ji*, the itching and pain had markedly diminished and his bowel movements were free and easy. Administration was stopped after 5 *ji* when the lesions had disappeared and the itching and pain had completely recovered.

"The Treatment of Herpes Zoster with *Xie Gan Ding Tong Tang* (Drain the Liver, Calm Pain Decoction)" by Wu Jin-mei & Chen Zhong-yi, *Shan Xi Zhong Yi (Shanxi Traditional Chinese Medicine)*, #5, 1993, p. 36; BF

This clinical audit describes the treatment of 32 cases of herpes zoster with *Xie Can Ding Tong Tang* in which this main formula was modified with additions and subtractions depending on the patients' pattern discrimination. Of the 32 cases, 23 were men and 9 were women. They ranged in age from 9-61 years of age with 25 being between 31-61. Seventeen cases had had this condition for 1 month, 12 for from 1-2 months, 2 for 3 months, and 1 for 8 months. In addition, 5 cases had lesions on their head and face, while 27 had lesions on their chest, abdomen, lateral costal region, or upper back.

Xie Gan Ding Tong Tang is composed of: Radix Gentianae Scabrae (*Long Dan Cao*), 10-15g, Fructus Gardeniae Jasminoidis (*Zhi Zi*), 10g, Radix Scutellariae Baicalensis (*Huang Qin*), 10g, Radix Bupleuri (*Chai Hu*), 10g, Radix Rehmanniae (*Sheng Di*), 12-20g, Rhizoma Corydalis Yanhusuo (*Yuan Hu*), 15g, Rhizoma Alismatis (*Ze Xie*), 20g, Radix Salviae Miltiorrhizae (*Dan Shen*), 30g, Radix Rubrus Paeoniae Lactiflorae (*Chi Shao*), 15g, Radix Albus Paeoniae Lactiflorae (*Bai Shao*), raw Radix Glycyrrhizae (*Sheng Gan Cao*), 6g, raw Concha Ostreae (*Sheng Mu Li*), 20g, raw Os Draconis (*Sheng Long Gu*), 20g, Concha Margaritiferae (*Zhen Zhu Mu*), 30g, Scolopendra Subspinipes (*Wu Gong*), 2 pieces, and Buthus Martensis (*Quan Xie*), 6g.

If the blisters had broken and were weeping a watery discharge accompanied by torpid intake, abdominal distention, and a white, slimy tongue coating indicating flourishing dampness, Caulis Akebiae Mutong (*Mu Tong*), Semen Plantaginis (*Che Qian Zi*), Rhizoma Atractylodis (*Cang Zhu*), Cortex Magnoliae Officinalis (*Hou Pu*), etc. were added. If the skin lesions were red and there was burning hot pain indicating flourishing heat, Herba Cum Radice Taraxaci Mongolici (*Pu Gong Ying*), Rhizoma Paridis Polyphyllae (*Zao Xiu*), Flos Chrysanthemi Indici (*Ye Ju Hua*), etc. were added. If the course of the disease had been prolonged, quickening the blood and transforming stasis medicinals were added, such as Semen Vaccariae Segetalis (*Wang Bu Liu Xing*), Rhizoma Ligustici Wallichii (*Chuan Xiong*), Semen Pruni Persicae (*Tao Ren*), Flos Carthami Tinctorii (*Hong Hua*), etc. One *ji* of

179

the above was decocted in water each day and taken in divided doses. All the patients treated with the above protocol were cured. Typically, improvement was seen with 1-2 *ji* with total cure occurring with 9-12 *ji*.

According to the authors, this condition is due either to a) internal damage by the emotions resulting in the flourishing of liver/-gallbladder fire, b) long-term spleen damp depression resulting in damp heat accumulating internally, or c) external invasion by toxic evils. However, damp heat is always the main distinguishing characteristic to which one's attention should be paid in the treatment of this condition. Therefore, this combination of medicinals have the functions of clearing heat and eliminating dampness, dispelling evils and stopping pain.

"61 Cases of Herpes Zoster Treated by *Chai Hu Qing Gan Tang* (Bupleurum Clear the Liver Decoction)" by Wang Pei-mao *et al.*, *Si Chuan Zhong Yi (Sichuan Traditional Chinese Medicine)*, #9, 1993, p. 37; BF

In this clinical audit, 36 cases of herpes zoster were treated with *Chai Hu Qing Gan Tang* with additions and subtractions. Of these 36, 17 were women and 19 were men. Their age ranged from a minimum of 15 to a maximum of 66 years of age. The shortest course of disease was 6 days and the longest was 15 days. The skin lesions were either red papules or watery blisters arranged in a belt-like row following nerve routes.These were accompanied by piercing pain.

The formula consisted of: Radix Bupleuri (*Chai Hu*), Rhizoma Ligustici Wallichii (*Chuan Xiong*), Radix Scutellariae Baicalensis (*Huang Qin*), and Fructus Gardeniae Jasminoidis (*Zhi Zi*), 9g @, Radix Albus Paeoniae Lactiflorae (*Bai Shao*), Radix Angelicae Sinensis (*Dang Gui*), Fructus Arctii Lappae (*Niu Bang Zi*), and Radix Trichosanthis Kirlowii (*Tian Hua Fen*), 12g @, Radix Rehmanniae (*Sheng Di*) and Fructus Forsythiae Suspensae (*Lian Qiao*), 15g @, and

Radix Ledebouriellae Sesloidis (*Fang Feng*) and Radix Glycyrrhizae (*Gan Cao*), 6g @. If heat toxins were heavy, Flos Lonicerae Japonicae (*Yin Hua*), Flos Chrysanthemi Indici (*Ye Ju Hua*), and Radix Isatidis Seu Baphicacanthi (*Ban Lang Gen*), 15g @, were added. If dampness was heavy, Rhizoma Atractylodis (*Cang Zhu*) and Cortex Phellodendri (*Huang Bai*), 12g @, and Radix Gentianae Scabrae (*Dan Cao*), 9g, were added. While if there was constipation, Radix Et Rhizoma Rhei (*Da Huang*), 9g, was added. These were decocted in water and taken, 1 *ji* per day, divided in two doses and taken warm.

All 36 patients were cured by taking the above formula and there was no recurrence of this condition on follow-up 3 months later. Six cases were healed after 7 days of the above herbs, 23 cases in from 7-14 days, and 7 cases healed in from 14-23 days. Typically, improvement was noted after taking 5 *ji*.

The authors describe the disease causes and mechanisms of this disease as being due to liver qi and depression binding transforming into fire and damp heat accumulating in the spleen channel simultaneously with infection by toxic evils. This then gives rise to an accumulation of damp heat fire toxins in the flesh and skin. *Chai Hu Qing Gan Tang* clears the liver and resolves depression, resolves toxins and disinhibits dampness, activates the blood and courses wind. Depending on the individual patient's pattern diagnosis, one should then emphasize either clearing liver heat, resolving toxic evils, of disinhibiting damp turbidity.

"A Short Discussion of the Treatment of 118 Cases of Herpes Zoster" by Tan Cheng-bang & Tan Mei-bang, *Jiang Xi Zhong Yi Yao (Jiangxi Traditional Chinese Medicine & Medicinals)*, #5, 1993, p. 27; BF

Besides giving the traditional Chinese medical names of this condition and describing the locations on the body most likely to exhibit lesions, *i.e.*, the chest and lateral costal regions, abdomen, upper back, head, and four extremities, they say that most cases of herpes heal in approximately 2 weeks and typically there is no recurrence. However, in the elderly or those with bodily vacuity, *i.e.*, constitutional weakness, there may be recurrent bouts or aching and pain lasting numerous weeks.

Of the 118 cases reported on in this study, 60 were men and 58 women. Fifteen cases were below 10 years of age, 30 cases were between 10-30, 73 cases were over 30 years of age. Forty-three cases healed within 7 days of treatment. While 75 cases healed in more than 7 days.

Two formulas were used. The first is called *Tu Ling He Ji* (Smilax Mixture). It consisted of: Rhizoma Smilacis Glabrae (*Tu Fu Ling*), Fructus Gardeniae Jasminoidis (*Zhi Zi*), Radix Scutellariae Baicalensis (*Huang Qin*), Cortex Phellodendri (*Huang Bai*), Herba Desmodii (*Jin Qian Cao*), and Herba Plantaginis (*Che Qian Cao*). The amounts of each ingredient used clinically was dependent on each patient's condition. If there was fever, Herba Cum Radice Taraxaci Mongolici (*Pu Gong Ying*) and Rhizoma Anemarrhenae (*Zhi Mu*) were added. If dampness was flourishing, Semen Coicis Lachryma-jobi (*Yi Yi Ren*) and Rhizoma Atractylodis (*Cang Zhu*) were added. If there was itching, Bombyx Batryticatus (*Jiang Can*) and Radix Sophorae Flavescentis (*Ku Shen*) were added. And if there was pain, Radix Albus Paeoniae Lactiflorae (*Bai Shao*) was added.

The second formula is called *Shao Gan Ci Zhe Tang* (Peony, Licorice, Magnetite, & Hematite Decoction). This formula was given specifically if there was nerve pain. It consisted of: Radix Albus Paeoniae Lactiflorae (*Bai Shao*), Radix Glycyrrhizae (*Gan Cao*), Magnetitum (*Ci Shi*), Haematitum (*Dai Zhe Shi*). Again the amounts of each ingredient was decided based on the patient's condition. If there was remaining toxins which had not been cleared, Fructus Gardeniae Jasminoidis (*Zhi Zi*), and Radix Scutellariae Baicalensis (*Huang Qin*) were added. If food and drink were less than normal, Massa Medica

Fermentata (*Jian Qu*) and Fructus Crataegi (*Shan Zha*) were added. If
there was constipation, Semen Cannabis Sativae (*Huo Ma Ren*) and Semen
Trichosanthis Kirlowii (*Gua Lou Ren*) were added. And if there was
bodily vacuity, Radix Astragali Membranacei (*Huang Qi*) and Radix
Glehniae Littoralis (*Sha Shen*) were added. In this study, 15 cases were
given this formula for post-herpetic neuralgia and all were cured.

"A Survey of the Combined Western & Traditional Chinese Medical Treatment of 320 Cases of Herpes Zoster" by Zhang Qing-hao & Zhang Geng-sheng, *Zhong Guo Zhong Xi Yi Jie He Za Zhi (The Chinese Journal of Integrated Chinese-Western Medicine)*, #11, 1993, p. 695; BF

This survey reports on the treatment of 320 cases of herpes zoster with
a combination of modern Western and Traditional Chinese Medicines.
Of the 320 cases, 198 were men and 122 were women. Four cases
were 10 years old, 185 cases were between 18-40, 85 cases were
between 41-60, and 46 cases were between 61-75 years of age.
Twenty-seven had herpes on their head and neck regions, 169 on their
chest and rib regions, 68 on their upper backs, 34 on their lower back
and abdominal regions, 12 on their upper extremities, and 10 on their
lower extremities. Characteristically, most of the lesions were
distributed along the intercostal and trigeminal nerves. The course of
disease (*i.e.*, the acute outbreak of lesions) ranged from as short as 3
days to as long as 13 days.

The method of treatment consisted of a modern Western medical
treatment and a traditional Chinese medical treatment. The modern
Western medical treatment used 2% lidocaine combined with vitamin
B_{12} introduced as a subdermal block at the site of the lesions. This was
done 1 time per day. The amount of the block was dependent on the
size of the lesion and was not fixed. The purpose of this treatment was

to diminish the aching and pain and to prevent the disease from spreading.

The Traditional Chinese Medicine treatment consisted of the use of self-composed formula called *Qing Zi Fang* (Green Purple Formula or Indigo & Lithospermum Formula). The formula's ingredients were: Pulvis Levis Indigonis (*Qing Dai*), 10g, Radix Lithospermi Seu Arnebiae (*Zi Cao*), 10g, Pulvis Calaminae (*Lu Gan Shi Fen*), 10g, stir-fried Semen Vaccariae Segetalis (*Chao Wang Bu Liu Xing*), 10g, Borneol (*Bing Pian*), 2g, and rice vinegar (*Mi Cu*), 100ml. The Lithospermum, Vaccariae, and Borneol were ground into fine powders and mixed with the Indigo and Calamine powders. The vinegar was then added to form a thin paste. This was then kept in a sealed container for future use. This paste was applied to the skin lesions enough to cover their surface to a depth of 0.2cm. The plasters were then covered with adhesive tape and the medicinals were changed 1 time per day.

Complete cure was defined as disappearance of the herpetic lesions and their attendant symptoms, scab formation or the falling off of any scabs formed. Good results were defined a reduction in the herpes lesions and their attendant symptoms, partial scab formation, or scabs falling off part of the lesions. No results were defined as no change in the herpes lesions and their attendant symptoms from before the treatment to after. Based on these criteria, all 320 cases experienced complete cure. The number of treatments varied from a high of 4 treatments to a low of 2, with the average being 3. Obvious improvement in the symptoms typically was seen within 24 hours. After 1 treatment, aching and pain was reduced and blisters began to shrivel. After 2 treatments, blisters dried up and formed scabs and any symptoms disappeared by themselves.

The authors state that herpes zoster is due to the herpes virus. It is seen mostly in older persons and is frequently accompanied by post-herpetic neuralgia. The above protocol combining Traditional Chinese and modern Western medicines gets a good results in a short course of treatment with a high cure rate and no sequelae. This disease is mostly due to heart/liver fire and heat, lung/spleen damp heat binding internally, and recurrent invasion by toxic evils. These mutually wrestle in the interstices of the flesh and obstruct the channels and connecting vessels with qi and blood not flowing freely.

This treatment clears heat and resolves toxins, eliminates dampness and engenders new flesh, and quickens the blood and stops pain. Within this formula (*i.e.*, the TCM formula), Indigo and Lithospermum clear heat, drain fire, and resolve toxins, cool the blood and scatter swelling. According to modern medical theory, Indigo and Lithospermum have antimicrobial and antiviral properties. Calamine and Borneol eliminate dampness and engender (new) flesh, disperse swelling and stop pain. While Vaccaria moves into the blood *fen* or level where it helps the blood move and not stop, run and not abide. It quickens the blood, disperses swelling, and stops pain. Thus taken as a whole, this formula has the power to clear heat, drain fire, and resolve toxins, eliminate dampness and engender flesh, and quicken the blood and stop pain.

"A Survey of the Treatment of Herpes Zoster with Cupping & Chinese Medicinals" by Li Zhen-hua, *Tian Jin Zhong Yi (Tianjin Traditional Chinese Medicine)*, #5, 1993, p. 36; BF

This study compares the treatment of 30 cases of herpes zoster with internally and externally administered Chinese medicinals and 60 cases treated with a combination of internal and external Chinese medicinals and cupping applied externally. There were 37 men and 53 women in this study. The patients ranged in age from 16-73 years old. The course of disease ranged from 2 days to 3 whole months. Fifty-two cases had had herpes lesions from 2 days-1 month, 21 from 1-2 months, and 13 for 3 whole months. All the cases had erythematous herpes lesions, scorching hot aching and pain, yellowish white water blisters or bloody blisters which easily burst and ulcerated discharging water. The aching and pain was lancinating and hard to bear. Their tongues were red with a yellow coating or were dark and purplish. Their pulses were wiry and slippery or wiry and rapid.

All 90 of the patients received two medicinal preparations for internal administration. The first was *Dan Cao Chong Ji* (Gentiana Soluble Granules): Radix Gentianae Scabrae (*Long Dan Cao*), Rhizoma Smilacis Glabrae (*Tu Fu Ling*), Herba Artemisiae Capillaris (*Yin Chen*), Radix Bupleuri (*Chai Hu*), Radix Scutellariae Baicalensis (*Huang Qin*), Fructus Gardeniae Jasminoidis (*Zhi Zi*), Rhizoma Alismatis (*Ze Xie*), raw Radix Rehmanniae (*Sheng Di*), Radix Angelicae Sinensis (*Dang Gui*), Semen Pruni Persicae (*Tao Ren*), Flos Carthami Tinctorii (*Hong Hua*), and Radix Glycyrrhizae (*Gan Cao*). The second was *Fu Zheng Xiao Du Yin* (Support the Righteous, Disperse Toxins Drink): Flos Chrysanthemi Indici (*Ye Ju Hua*), Flos Lonicerae Japonicae (*Yin Hua*), Fructus Forsythiae Suspensae (*Lian Qiao*), Herba Cum Radice Taraxaci Mongolici (*Pu Gong Ying*), Herba Violae Yedoensis (*Di Ding*), Radix Astragali Membranacei (*Huang Qi*), and Radix Angelicae Sinensis (*Dang Gui*). Each of these preparations were administered 1 time per day. All the patients also received daily applications of *Huan Wu Gan Shuang* (Circling Crow Glucoside Powder, a patent medicine).

In addition to the above, 60 patients in the so-called treatment group received cupping therapy. This consisted of first disinfecting the lesions with 75% ethyl alcohol. After disinfection, the area was pricked with a three-edged needle. If there were water blisters, these were broken and their fluid was discharged. If there were no water blisters, the erythematous area or the area which felt painful was pricked to break the skin and to let out blood. Then the area was cupped with the cups left in place for 15 minutes. When the cups were removed, they removed with them blister fluid and static blood. This was followed by the application of *Huan Wu Gan Shuang*. This method was repeated 1 time per day.

Cure consisted of the complete disappearance of the aching and pain, drying up and shrivelling of the blisters, and falling off of any scabs. Marked improvement consisted of obvious diminishment of the aching and pain or only slight aching, drying and shrivelling of the blisters, and falling off of any scabs. Some improvement consisted of diminishment of the aching and pain and drying and shrivelling of some of the blisters. Based on these criteria, of the 60 patients who received both the internal and external treatments, 27 cases or 45% were cured, 15 cases or 25% were markedly improved, 11 cases or 18.3% had some improvement, and 7 cases or 11.7% had no result. This yielded a combined amelioration rate of 88.3%. In the so-called control group which only received the internal medication and the application of the *Huan Wu Gan Shuang*, 2 cases or 6.7% were cured, 8 cases or 26.7% experienced marked improvement, 3 cases or 10% experienced some improvement, and 17 cases or 56.6% experienced no improvement. Thus, in the control group, the amelioration rate was only 43.3%. This suggests that cupping therapy administered with internal and external Chinese herbal therapy is twice as effective for herpes zoster as Chinese herbal therapy alone.

Facial Acne

"The Treatment of 123 Cases of Facial Acne" by Xu Jian-ping, *Jiang Su Zhong Yi (Jiangsu Traditional Chinese Medicine)*, #12, 1992, p. 17; BF

This research report describes the treatment of 123 cases of facial acne. Of these 123 cases, 81 were men and 42 were women. The youngest was 16 years old and the oldest was 48 with most of the patients falling between 18-35 years of age. The shortest duration of this disease was 1/2 month, the longest was 8 years, and the average was 3.6 years. Treatment was given on the basis of a pattern discrimination

1. Lung channel wind heat (77 cases)

The acne of patients categorized as suffering from lung channel wind heat consisted of raised, red colored lesions scattered around the face approximately the size of grains of millet. Some of these raised lesions or pimples had small, pussy heads and occasionally ached and were painful. This was accompanied by a thirsty mouth with a preference for cold drinks. The stools were dry and bound and the urination was frequent and red. The tongue had a thin, yellow coating and the pulse was rapid.

Rx: Cortex Radicis Mori Albi (*Sang Bai Pi*), Folium Eriobotryae (*Pi Pa Ye*), Cortex Phellodendri (*Huang Bai*), Rhizoma Anemarrhenae (*Zhi Mu*), Radix Et Rhizoma Rhei (*Sheng Chuan Jun*), Fructus Forsythiae Suspensae (*Lian Qiao*), Radix Glycyrrhizae (*Sheng Gan Cao*), 10g @, Rhizoma Coptidis Chinensis (*Chuan Lian*), 5g, Herba Oldenlandiae Diffusae (*She She Cao*), 30g

2. Heat & stasis binding together (31 cases)

These patients' acne consisted of raised lesions or pimples on the face which were colored dark red and approximately the size of beans. Under pressure, they felt hard and bound or knotted and were cyst-like. There was swelling and pain or after rupturing there was a small amount of pussy matter secretion. If the skin was injured, the hair (follicular) holes or openings increased in width and there were blackheads. Afterwards, they remained sunken or became indented scars. The tongue had ecchymotic spots and the pulse was astringent/choppy.

Rx: Radix Angelicae Sinensis (*Dang Gui*), Radix Rubrae Paeoniae Lactiflorae (*Chi Shao*), 12g @, Flos Carthami Tinctorii (*Hong Hua*), Semen Pruni Persicae (*Tao Ren*), Rhizoma Ligustici Wallichii (*Chuan*

Xiong), Radix Bupleuri (*Chai Hu*), blackened Fructus Gardeniae Jasminoidis (*Hei Shan Zhi*), 10g @, Concha Ostreae (*Mu Li*), 30g, Herba Violae Yedoensis (*Di Ding Cao*), 15g

3. Yin vacuity, fire effulgent (15 cases)

In this group, the raised lesions or pimples were fine and small, approximately the size of grains of rice. Their color was dark red accompanied by scant or minor possible nodulation with no pus secretion. After rupturing, a small amount of white colored secretion appeared like smashed rice. This was accompanied by a tidal or flushed red facial color, a dry mouth and heart vexation, diminished sleep and excessive dreams, low back and knee soreness and weakness, a red tongue with scant coating, and a fine and rapid pulse.

Rx: Fructus Tribuli Terrestris (*Bai Ji Li*), Herba Artemisiae Apiaceae (*Qing Hao*), Radix Glycyrrhizae (*Sheng Gan Cao*), 10g @, Radix Scrophulariae Ningpoensis (*Xuan Shen*), Cortex Radicis Lycii (*Di Gu Pi*), Cortex Radicis Moutan (*Dan Pi*), Radix Rubrus Paeoniae Lactiflorae (*Chi Shao*), 12g @, Radix Rehmanniae (*Sheng Di*), 15g, Rhizoma Coptidis Chinensis (*Chuan Lian*), 5g

According to the author, no matter what the above pattern discrimination, one can use (the following modifications with any of the above guiding formulas): If the face has an excessively oily secretion, add Folium Mori Albi (*Sang Ye*) and Fructus Crataegi (*Sheng Shan Zha*). If the skin lesions itch, add Cortex Radicis Dictamni (*Bai Xian Pi*) and Radix Kochiae (*Di Fu Zi*). If heat is predominant, add double the amount of Flos Lonicerae Japonicae (*Yin Hua*) and Herba Violae Yedoensis (*Di Ding*, measuring by) *liang*. If there is hard, difficult to dissipate nodulation, one can take *Nei Xiao Pian* (Internal Dispersing Tablets). If there is qi vacuity, add Radix Astragali Membranacei (*Sheng Huang Qi*). While taking these herbs internally, apply at the same time *Zi Dian Dao San* (Child Crown Collapse Powder) or *Fu*

Yan Ding (Skin Inflammation Tincture) to the affected areas.

Complete cure consisted of complete disappearance of the skin lesions with no recurrence within 1/2 year. Marked improvement consisted of disappearance of 70% or more of the skin lesions. Fair improvement consisted of 30% or more disappearance of skin lesions or disappearance but subsequent reappearance after the herbs were discontinued. Of the 77 cases suffering from lung channel wind heat, 49 were cured, 22 experienced marked improvement, 5 fair improvement, and 1 experienced no result. Of the 31 cases of heat and stasis, 12 were cured, 12 had marked improvement, 7 fair improvement, and 2 no result. And of the 15 cases of yin vacuity, fire effulgent, 7 were cured, 3 experienced marked improvement, 4 fair improvement, and 1 no result. Thus of the 123 cases total, 68 cases (53.7%) experienced complete cure, 37 (30.1%) marked improvement, 16 (13.0%) fair improvement, and 4 (3.4%) no result. Further, among the 68 cases that were cured, the length of administration was between 27 days and 3 months. Most showed signs of improvement in their skin lesions within 7-10 days. If, after 1/2 month of taking the above herbs, there was no result, these patients were categorized as receiving no result and the herbs were discontinued.

Polymorphous Sunlight Eruptions

"The Treatment of 20 Cases of Polymorphous Sunlight Eruptions with the Chinese Medicinals, *Fu Ji Pi Yan Xi Fang* (Recurrent Seasonal Dermatitis Wash Formula)" by Xi Wen-wang, *Zhong Guo Zhong Xi Yi Jie He Za Zhi (The Chinese Journal of Integrated Chinese-Western Medicine)*, #11, 1993, p. 695-6; BF

This survey reports on the treatment of polymorphous sunlight eruptions using an external wash made from Chinese medicinals. Of the 20 cases, 5 were men and 15 were women. Their ages ranged from a low of 16 to a high of 80 years of age, with 18 cases between 20-40 years of age. Eighteen cases had had this disease for less than 3 months and 2 for more than 3 months. All 20 of these patients used _Fu Ji Pi Yan Xi Fang_ as an externally applied wash. They were also allowed to simultaneously use at their own discretion other externally applied herbal materials treatments.

Fu Ji Pi Yan Xi Fang consists of: Flos Lonicerae Japonicae (_Yin Hua_), 30g, Herba Cum Radice Taraxaci Mongolici (_Pu Gong Ying_), 15g, Radix Ledebouriellae Sesloidis (_Fang Feng_), 12g, Fructus Arctii (_Niu Bang Zi_), 15g, Herba Menthae (_Bo He_), 6g, Cortex Radicis Dictamni (_Bai Xian Pi_), 15g, Fructus Kochiae Scopariae (_Di Fu Zi_), 15g, Radix Sophorae Flavescentis (_Ku Shen_), 10g, Radix Lithospermi Seu Arnebiae (_Zi Cao_), 15g, Cortex Radicis Moutan (_Dan Pi_), 10g, and raw Radix Glycyrrhizae (_Sheng Gan Cao_), 6g.

If there was redness, swelling, heat, and pain, Folium Isatidis (_Da Qing Ye_) and Flos Chrysanthemi Indici (_Ye Ju Hua_) were added. If there was copious oozing and weeping, Rhizoma Atractylodis (_Cang Zhu_) and Herba Polygoni Avicularis (_Bian Xu_) were added. And if there was itching, Herba Equiseti Hiemalis (_Mu Zei_) was added. These medicinals were placed in 1500ml of water and decocted for 15 minutes. After they became warm, the affected area was washed with this decoction. This was done 2 times per day, using 1 _ji_ per day, with 5 _ji_ equalling one complete course of treatment.

Complete cure was defined as complete disappearance of the skin lesions and stopping of any itching. Improvement was defined as reduction of the skin lesions and diminishment of itching. No result was defined as no obvious change in the skin lesions after 1 course of treatment with itching either not reduced or increased. Based on these criteria, 12 cases or 60% experienced complete cure. Six cases or 30% experienced improvement. And 2 cases or 10% got no results.

The smallest number of herbs used was 1 *ji* and the largest was 8 *ji* with the average being 4.9 *ji*.

According to the author, polymorphous sunlight eruptions have no clear cause. This condition tends to get worse in spring and summer and decreases in winter and fall. Traditional Chinese Medicine regards this condition as being due to an innate disposition with recurrent invasion of wind heat evils, lack of spleen movement and transportation, and damp heat engendered internally. This becomes depressed in the flesh and skin and results in these eruptions. *Fu Ji Pi Yan Xi Fang* clears heat and disinhibits dampness. Lonicera, Taraxacum, Dictamnus, and raw Licorice clear heat and resolve toxins. Lithospermum and Moutan clear heat and cool the blood. Kochia and Sophora Flavescens clear heat and disinhibit dampness, while Ledebouriella, Arctium, and Mint dispel wind and scatter heat.

Psoriasis

"The Treatment of 51 Cases of Psoriasis with *Jie Du Huo Xue Tang* (Resolve Toxins, Quicken the Blood Decoction)" by Liu Shi-li, Fang Bing, & Zhang Zuo-zhou, *Zhong Yi Za Zhi (Journal of Traditional Chinese Medicine)*, #9, 1993, p. 549-50; BF

The authors begin this report by stating that psoriasis is a commonly encountered chronic skin disease making up between 5-10% of the patients in a dermatology out-patient clinic. Based on the Chinese medical principles of clearing heat and resolving toxins, quickening the blood and dispelling wind, the authors composed the formula *Jie Du Huo Xue Tang* for the treatment of psoriasis which they then used to treat 51 cases of this disease.

Of the 51, 26 were men and 25 were women. They ranged in age from 8.5-66 years of age. Forty-seven had ordinary psoriasis, 1 had secondary psoriasis, 2 had psoriasis with erythroderma, and 2 had articular psoriasis (one of which also had erythroderma). The course of disease had lasted as short as 1 month and as long as 47 years. Forty-seven cases had been treated previously with various Western medications and Chinese herbal medicine, including externally applied plasters.

Jie Du Huo Xue Tang consists of: Herba Cum Radice Taraxaci Mongolici (*Pu Gong Ying*), Radix Isatidis Seu Baphicacanthi (*Ban Lang Gen*), Rhizoma Paridis Polyphyllae (*Zao Xiu*), Herba Oldenlandiae (*Bai Hua She She Cao*), Rhizoma Sparganii (*San Leng*), Rhizoma Curcumae Zedoariae (*E Zhu*), Fructus Tribuli Terrestris (*Bai Ji Li*), and Herba Solani Nigri (*Long Kui*).

Based on a pattern discrimination, if there was severe blood heat with bright red skin lesions, Rhizoma Imperatae Cylindricae (*Mao Gen*) and raw Radix Rehmanniae (*Sheng Di*) were added. If wind was flourishing and itching was severe, Zaocys Dhumnades (*Wu She*) and Bombyx Batryticatus (*Jang Can*) were added. If wind and dampness were obstructing the connecting vessels with joint *bi* pain, Herba Gentianae Macrophyllae (*Qin Jiao*) and Cortex Radicis Dictamni (*Bai Xian Pi*) were added. If blood dryness was damaging yin with dry, parched skin lesions and large scales, Radix Angelicae Sinensis (*Dang Gui*), Radix Salviae Miltiorrhizae (*Dan Shen*), and Fructus Ligustri Lucidi (*Nu Zhen Zi*) were added. One *ji* was used per day, decocted in water and taken in two doses. Four weeks equalled 1 complete course of treatment. If there was no cure after a single course, from 2-4 courses were given. The patients were examined again once every 1-2 weeks. During the course of treatment, twenty-four patients had blood and urine tests and their liver functions assessed. Also, during the above treatment, patients were not allowed to use any other medications.

Of the 51 patients, 26 or 51% were clinically cured. Twenty-two or

43.1% experienced improvement. And 3 cases or 5.9% experienced no result. Of the 11 cases with a disease duration of 1 year or less, 6 cases were cured and 5 were improved. Of the 12 cases with a disease duration of 1-5 years, 4 were cured and 8 were improved. Of the 10 cases with this disease 6-10 years, 6 were cured and 4 were improved. Of the 18 cases who had suffered for 11 years or more, 9 were cured, 6 improved, and 3 got no results. The shortest duration of treatment was 2 weeks and the longest was 6 whole courses of treatment, with most cases receiving between 2-3 courses. Among those that were cured, 3 had relapses which were cured after another course of treatment. No abnormal changes were found in the 24 cases who had had their blood and urine tested and liver functions assessed and there were no obvious side effects to this treatment.

Lower Leg Ulcers

"A Survey of the Treatment of 50 Cases of Lower Leg Ulcers with *Zhu Fan San* (Margarita & Alum Powder)" by Zhao Ming-li *et al.*, *Zhong Yi Za Zhi (The Journal of Traditional Chinese Medicine)*, #9, 1993, p. 551-2; BF

The treatment of ulcers on the lower legs with Western medicine is not usually satisfactory and the condition tends to recur. Therefore, between Oct. 1990 and Oct. 1991, the authors of this survey treated 50 cases of lower leg ulcers with a self-composed formula named *Zhu Fan San*. Of the 50 cases, 16 were treated as outpatients and 34 were treated in the hospital. Thirty-one were men and 19 were women. Their ages ranged from a high of 85 to a low of 18 years old, with the average being 60. Two cases were less than 30, 15 were between 30-50, and 33 were over 50 years old. Sixteen cases had accompanying conditions. Of these, 7 had diabetes mellitus, 5 eczema, and 4 high blood pressure. As for causes, 41 cases were due to venous problems, 7 were due to external injury, and 2 were due to infected incisions.

The course of disease ranged from as long as 50 years to as short as 10 days. And the ulcers themselves were from as small as 1cm x 1cm to as large as 20cm x 10cm, with 36 cases or 60% being larger than 2cm x 2cm.

Zhu Fan San is composed of: Radix Pseudoginseng (_San Qi_), 10g, Alum (_Ku Fan_), 10g, Borneol (_Bing Pian_), 10g, and Margarita (_Zhen Zhu_), 10g. These were ground, sifted through a 200 "eye" screen, and packed in a bottle to be stored for use. Prior to using this powder, the ulcers were disinfected with ethyl alcohol and allowed to dry. The powder was applied to the mouth of the wound, the amount of the powder depending on the size of the ulcer. The typical rate was 2-4g/cm^2. However, this medicated powder should not applied too thickly. This dressing was cleaned and reapplied 1-2 times per day. If there were accompanying conditions, these were treated by clearing heat and resolving toxins, quickening the blood and transforming stasis, opening the connecting vessels and disinhibiting medicinals taken orally, such as Flos Lonicerae Japonicae (_Yin Hua_), Fructus Forsythiae Suspensae (_Lian Qiao_), Herba Cum Radice Taraxaci Mongolici (_Pu Gong Ying_), Herba Violae Yedoensis (_Di Ding Cao_), Radix Rubrus Paeoniae Lactiflorae (_Chi Shao_), Cortex Radicis Moutan (_Dan Pi_), Cortex Sclerotii Rubri Poriae Cocos (_Chi Ling Pi_), Rhizoma Alismatis (_Ze Xie_), etc., 7-10 _ji_.

Cure consisted of healing of the ulcer with complete disappearance of symptoms. If the ulcers became smaller by more than 50% and the clinical symptoms disappeared, this was defined as improvement. Treatment lasted from as long as 87 days to as short as 5 days, with the average being 28 days. Forty-eight cases were completely cured and 2 cases were improved. Thus the combined amelioration rate was 100% and the cure rate was 96%.

Case history: Male, 65 years of age. The patient had had phlebitis in both lower legs for 9 years. He had several ulcers on both of his lower legs, the largest of which was 10cm x 8cm by 0.5cm deep. The ulcers were dark red and exuded a yellow fluid. Both lower legs also exhibited pitting edema. The patient's tongue was purple with a yellow coating and his pulse was slippery and rapid. His white blood cell count was 7600/mm³ and blood sugar was negative. His pattern discrimination was damp heat pouring downward with toxic heat obstructing the connecting vessels. Besides being treated with *Zhu Fan San* above, he was also administered orally Flos Lonicerae Japonicae (*Yin Hua*), 30g, Fructus Forsythiae Suspensae (*Lian Qiao*), 20g, Herba Cum Radice Taraxaci Mongolici (*Pu Gong Ying*), 15g, Herba Violae Yedoensis (*Di Ding Cao*), 15g, Cortex Sclerotii Rubri Poriae Cocos (*Chi Ling Pi*), 15g, Rhizoma Alismatis (*Ze Xie*), 15g, Caulis Akebiae Mutong (*Mu Tong*), 10g, Semen Plantaginis (*Che Qian Zi*), 10g, Radix Rubrus Paeoniae Lactiflorae (*Chi Shao*), 12g, Cortex Radicis Moutan (*Dan Pi*), 12g, Rhizoma Ligustici Wallichii (*Chuan Xiong*), 12g, and Caulis Millettiae Seu Spatholobi (*Ji Xue Teng*), 20g. He was given 14 *ji*. Sixteen days later, the ulcer had begun to close and the edema of the lower extremities was dispersed. Twenty days later, the right leg had healed completely and the left leg had one ulcer 1.5cm x 1cm and another 3cm x 1 cm. With treatment, 38 days later he was completely cured.

Bedsores

"The Treatment of 96 Cases of Bedsores with *Sheng Ji San* (Engender Flesh Powder)" by Xu Jin-mu & Wang Zhe-zhong, *He Nan Zhong Yi (Henan Traditional Chinese Medicine)*, #9, 1993, p. 230; BF

Since 1988, the authors have treated 96 cases of bedsores with their self-composed *Sheng Ji San*. This formula consists of: processed Calamina (*Zhi Lu Gan Shi*), 15g, Stalactitum (*Di Ru Shi*), 9g, Talcum (*Hua Shi*), 30g, Succinum (*Xue Po*), 9g, Cinnabaris (*Zhu Sha*), 3g, and Borneol (*Bing Pian*), 0.3g. These were ground into a fine powder and packed in a bottle for future use. According to the authors, this formula functions to eliminate dampness and close sores, engender flesh and contract openings. After disinfecting the sore, this powder was applied over the open wound. Ninety-four cases were cured by this treatment and 2 cases experienced no result. Thus the amelioration rate was 97.92%.

Facial Flat Warts

"The Treatment of 56 Cases of Facial Flat Warts with Self-composed *Qu You Fang* (Eliminate Warts Formula)" by Ma Shao-wu & Zhou Dong, *Shang Hai Zhong Yi Yao Za Zhi (The Shanghai Journal of Traditional Chinese Medicine & Medicinals)*, #9, 1993, p. 28; BF

According to the authors, flat warts are a commonly seen dermatological condition for which there is as yet no exceptionally effective (Western) medicinals. Therefore, the authors have composed a Chinese medicinal treatment for this condition called *Qu You Fang*. Of the 56 cases the authors report on treating with this protocol, 16 were males and 40 were females. The youngest aged was 10 and the oldest was 64, with 48 cases aged between 21-30. Eight cases had had this condition for from 1-6 months, 20 cases for from 6 months-1 year, 10 cases from 1-2 years, 12 cases from 2-3 years, and 6 cases for more than 3 years. Ten cases had more than 100 warts, while 46 cases had less than 100.

Qu You Fang was prescribed on the basis of TCM pattern discrimination. The formula's uses are to clear heat and resolve toxins, quicken the blood and dispel stasis, soften the hard and scatter nodulation. The formula is comprised of: Herba Portulacae Oleraceae (*Ma Chi Xian*), 30g, Radix Isatidis Seu Baphicacanthi (*Ban Lang Gen*), 30g, raw

Semen Coicis Lachryma-jobi (*Sheng Mi Ren*), 30g, Radix Lithospermi Seu Arnebiae (*Zi Cao*), 9g, Flos Chrysanthemi Indici (*Ye Ju Hua*), 9g, Flos Lonicerae Japonicae (*Yin Hua*), 9g, Rhizoma Paridis Polyphyllae (*Zao Xiu*), 15g, Herba Oldenlandiae (*Bai Hua She She Cao*), 30g, Semen Pruni Persicae (*Tao Ren*), Flos Carthami Tinctorii (*Hong Hua*), 9g, mix-fried Squama Manitis (*Zhi Shan Jia*), 9g, mix-fried Bombyx Batryticatus (*Zhi Jiang Can*), 9g, raw Os Draconis (*Sheng Long Gu*, decocted in advance), 30g, raw Concha Ostreae (*Sheng Mu Li*, decocted in advance), 30g.

If the disease had lasted a long time and there was qi and blood dual vacuity symptoms, Radix Astragali Membranacei (*Huang Qi*), 30g, and Radix Salviae Miltiorrhizae (*Dan Shen*), 9g, were added. If there was itching, Cortex Radicis Dictamni (*Bai Xian Pi*), 30g, and Herba Equiseti Hiemalis (*Mu Zei Cao*), 12g, were added. If the warts were hard and tough, Spica Prunellae Vulgaris (*Xia Gu Cao*), 15g, Thallus Algae (*Kun Bu*), 9g, and Herba Sargassii (*Hai Zao*), 9g, were added.

The above medicinals were soaked in 500ml of water for 45 minutes (the precooked medicinals having already been decocted for 30 minutes). Then more water was added and the medicinals were decocted for another 15 minutes. After decoction, 300ml of liquid was poured off and taken in 2 divided doses. These medicinals were decocted a second time for 10 minutes after again adding more water, resulting in 500ml of liquid. This was divided into several doses and the warts were rubbed and washed with this decoction. After that, they were scraped with a knife. This resulted in the skin becoming scorching hot but not injured. Each day 1 *ji* was used and 3 whole months equalled 1 course of treatment.

Cure was defined as complete disappearance of the warts. Their reduction by more than 70% was defined as marked improvement. Some improvement was defined as approximately 30% reduction of the warts. And no result meant that there was no change in the patient's condition after 3 months of the above treatment. Of the 56 people treated, 30 experienced cure, 12 marked improvement, 8 some improvement, and 6 no result. This yielded a combined amelioration rate of 89.3%. The shortest course of treatment was 1 day and the longest was 3 whole months. Most cases that were healed did so within 30-60 days.

Hypersensitive Chronic Lip Inflammation

"The Pattern Discrimination Herbal Medicine Treatment of 35 Cases of Hypersensitive Chronic Lip Inflammation" by Lai Zong-yu, _Si Chuan Zhong Yi (Sichuan Traditional Chinese Medicine)_, #10, 1993, p. 43; BF

In Traditional Chinese Medicine, this condition is called lip wind and lip dry cracking. Between July 1984 and October 1990, the author had occasion to treat 35 cases of this condition using pattern discrimination with good results. Of the 35 cases, 13 were men and 22 were women. Three were under 25 years of age, 18 were between 25-40, and 14 were between 41-55. The longest course of disease was 8 years and the shortest was 2 years.

1. Spleen & stomach damp heat pattern (16 cases)

The symptoms these patients manifested were cracked, chapped lips, ulcers with either pussy blood or a fluid discharge, bad breath, thirst but no desire to drink, constipation, reddish (_i.e._, dark), hot urination, a red tongue with a thick, yellow, slimy coating, and a slippery, rapid pulse. In this case, the treatment principles were to clear the spleen and drain heat, disinhibit dampness and resolve toxins using _Qing Pi Chu Shi Yin Jia Jian_ (Clear the Spleen, Eliminate Dampness Drink with Additions & Subtractions): raw Radix Rehmanniae (_Sheng Di_), Radix Scutellariae Baicalensis (_Huang Qin_), Sclerotium Poriae Cocos (_Fu Ling_), Rhizoma Atractylodis Macrocephalae (_Bai Zhu_), Rhizoma

Atractylodis (*Cang Zhu*), Fructus Gardeniae Jasminoidis (*Zhi Zi*), Cortex Radicis Moutan (*Dan Pi*), Tuber Ophiopogonis Japonicae (*Mai Dong*), Rhizoma Alismatis (*Ze Xie*), and Herba Artemisiae Capillaris (*Yin Chen*), 12g @, and Radix Glycyrrhizae (*Gan Cao*), 6g.

2. Yin vacuity harboring dampness pattern (8 cases)

The symptoms this group of patients manifested were heart vexation and easy anger, thirst, dry throat, repeated recurrence of sores and ulcers, chapped lips, oozing of fluids and bleeding, a red tongue with yellow coating, and a fine, rapid pulse. The treatment principles in this case were to nourish yin, clear heat, and disinhibit dampness using *Zhi Bai Di Huang Tang Jia Jian* (Anemarrhena & Phellodendron Rehmannia Decoction with Additions & Subtractions): raw Radix Rehmanniae (*Sheng Di*), Radix Trichosanthis Kirlowii (*Hua Fen*), Rhizoma Anemarrhenae (*Zhi Mu*), Cortex Phellodendri (*Huang Bai*), Tuber Ophiopogonis Japonicae (*Mai Dong*), Fructus Ligustri Lucidi (*Nu Zhen*), Cortex Radicis Lycii (*Di Gu Pi*), Cortex Radicis Moutan (*Dan Pi*), and Fructus Lycii Chinensis (*Gou Qi Zi*), 12g @, Radix Scrophulariae Ningpoensis (*Xuan Shen*) and Radix Isatidis Seu Baphicacanthi (*Ban Lang Gen*), 15g @, and Radix Glycyrrhizae (*Gan Cao*), 6g.

3. Blood vacuity transforming into dryness pattern (11 cases)

These patients' symptoms included a pale, lusterless face, decreased food (intake), loose stools, dizziness and vertigo, shortness of breath, sluggish speech, chapped and cracked lips, possible bleeding from the cracks, dryness, itching, and scaling, a pale tongue with thin, white, slightly yellow coating, and a fine, weak pulse. In this case, the treatment principles were to boost the qi and strengthen the spleen, nourish the blood and moisten dryness using *Dang Gui Tang Jia Jian* (*Dang Gui* Decoction with Additions & Subtractions): Radix Codonopsis Pilosulae (*Dang Shen*) and Radix Astragali Membranacei (*Huang Qi*), 15g @, Rhizoma Atractylodis Macrocephalae (*Bai Zhu*), Sclerotium Poriae Cocos (*Fu Ling*), Radix Angelicae Sinensis (*Dang*

Gui), Rhizoma Ligustici Wallichii (_Chuan Xiong_), Radix Albus Paeoniae Lactiflorae (_Bai Shao_), raw Radix Rehmanniae (_Sheng Di_), Cortex Radicis Moutan (_Dan Pi_), 12g @, Radix Scutellariae Baicalensis (_Huang Qin_), 9g, and dry Rhizoma Zingiberis (_Gan Jiang_) and Radix Glycyrrhizae (_Gan Cao_), 6g @.

One _ji_ was decocted in water and administered per day, divided in 3 doses, with 6 days equalling 1 course of treatment. In addition, a 3% hydrogen peroxide solution was applied and allowed to dry. This was then followed by the application of aureomycin cream.

Complete cure consisted of healing of the lesions after not more than 3 courses of treatment with no recurrence within a half year. Marked results were defined as healing of the lesions within 3 courses of therapy. However, after discontinuing the medicinals, the sores returned as before. These were then eliminated when the treatment was repeated. Some results were defined as partial elimination of the sores after 3 courses of treatment. And no results meant just that. Based on these criteria, 23 cases or 65.7% were completely cured, 8 cases or 22.8% were markedly improved, 3 cases or 8.6% were somewhat improved, and 1 case or 2.85% got no results from this protocol. Therefore, the combined amelioration rate was 97.13%. Further breakdown by pattern showed that of the 16 cases of spleen/stomach damp heat, 12 were cured and 4 got marked improvement. Of the 8 cases of yin vacuity harboring dampness, 5 were cured, 2 were markedly improved, and 1 was somewhat improved. And of the 11 cases of blood vacuity transforming into dryness pattern, 6 were cured, 2 markedly improved, 2 somewhat improved, and 1 got no results.

In their concluding discussion, the author mainly relates this condition to the spleen and stomach. This is based on the saying that the spleen opens into the portal of the mouth and has its efflorescence in the lips. Therefore, this disease is mostly caused by _yang ming_ stomach channel wind fire overwhelming above and spleen channel blood dryness. Blood vacuity engenders wind and transforms into dryness which may consume and damage yin blood. Spleen/stomach damp heat may obstruct and accumulate or heat evils may damage yin resulting in yin vacuity and internal heat with the spleen losing its propulsion and movement, thus resulting in phlegm dampness being generated internally. Thus the treatment of this disease should mainly be aimed at the spleen.

Drinker's Nose (*i.e.*, Acne Rosacea)

"The Treatment of 39 Cases of Drinker's Nose Using *Ma Xing Gan Shi Tang* (Ephedra, Armeniaca, Licorice, & Gypsum Decoction) with Additions" by Zou Shi-guang, *Zhe Jiang Zhong Yi Za Zhi (The Zhejiang Journal of Traditional Chinese Medicine)*, 1993, p. 323; CC

In this clinical study, the author successfully used *Ma Xing Gan Shi Tang* with additions to treat drinker's nose. The prescription contained: Herba Ephedrae (*Ma Huang*), 6g, raw Radix Glycyrrhizae (*Sheng Gan Cao*), 6g, Gypsum (*Shi Gao*), 45g, Semen Pruni Armeniacae (*Xing Ren*), 10g, Radix Et Rhizoma Rhei (*Da Huang*), 4g, raw Radix Rehmanniae (*Da Sheng Di*), 30g, Herba Oldenlandiae Diffusae (*Bai Hua She She Cao*), 20g, and Herba Scutellariae Barbatae (*Ban Zhi Lian*), 15g. One *ji* was decocted 3 times per day. The first 2 decoctions were mixed and administered morning and evening. All 3 of the decoctions were also administered topically to the nasal area for 5 minutes at a time. Two weeks constituted 1 course of therapy, and the treatment typically required 1-3 courses. If the skin was dusky red, thickened, and unnecessarily raised and enlarged, then 20g each of Radix Paeoniae Rubri (*Chi Shao*) and Radix Salviae Miltiorrhizae (*Dan Shen*) were added.

Thirty-five cases showed marked improvement defined by the disappearance of the symptoms of redness, thickening of the skin, and papules. Four cases did not respond to this therapy.

Shang Gu Ke
Traumatology & Orthopedics _____

Fractured Ribs

"The Administration of Chinese Medicinals in the Treatment of 32 Cases of Fractured Ribs" by Feng Ji-chen, *Zhe Jiang Zhong Yi Za Zhi (The Zhejiang Journal of Traditional Chinese Medicine)*, #5, 1993, p. 207; CC

This study compares the treatment of two groups of patients with fractured ribs. One group, labelled the treatment group, received Chinese medicinals. The other group did not. This group was called the comparison group. The group receiving Chinese medicinals was administered two separate formulas, one during the early stage of injury characterized by pain and soreness and another during the late or healing stage.

Early Stage (pain and soreness)

Fu Yuan Huo Xue Tang Jia Jian (Return to the Origin Quicken the Blood Decoction with Additions & Subtractions): Radix Bupleuri (*Chai Hu*), 10-15g, Fructus Meliae Toosendan (*Chuan Lian Zi*), 10-15g, Lumbricus (*Di Long*), 10-15g, Radix Angelicae Sinensis (*Dang Gui*), 12g, Radix Et Rhizoma Rhei (*Da Huang*), 5-10g, Flos Carthami Tinctorii (*Hong Hua*), 9-12g, Semen Pruni Persicae (*Tao Ren*), 9-12g, Radix Trichosanthis Kirlowii (*Tian Hua Fen*), 9-12g, Radix Gentianae Macrophyllae (*Qin Jiao*), 20g, raw Radix Astragali Membranacei (*Sheng Huang Qi*), 15-30g, Radix Pseudoginseng (*Shen San Qi*, swallowed as a powder), 3g, Herba Cum Radice Asari Sieboldi (*Xi Xin*), 1-2g, and Radix Glycyrrhizae (*Gan Cao*), 4-6g.

Dosage is adjusted based on constitution, age, degree of pain, and the course of illness. One *ji* of the above medicinals was taken daily until the thoracic pain ceased completely.

Late Stage (healing stage)

Jie Gu II Hao Fang (Bone Knitting Formula #II with Additions): Radix Dipsaci (*Xu Duan*), 15g, Rhizoma Drynariae (*Gu Sui Bu*), 15g, Pyritum (*Zi Ran Tong*), 15-30g, Radix Rubrus Paeoniae Lactiflorae (*Chi Shao*), 15-30g, and Rhizoma Curcumae (*Jiang Huang*), 9-12g. The doses within this prescription are adjusted based upon the patient's constitution and the integrity of the transportative and transformative functions of the middle warmer. One *ji* of the above medicinals was administered daily until the ends of the fracture had completely healed.

In the comparison group, the overall pain and soreness disappeared within 21 days. The pain and soreness with cough and expectoration disappeared within 36 days. And the bone break was healed within 45 days. In the group treated with the above Chinese medicinals, the overall pain and soreness disappeared within 7 days. The pain and soreness with cough and expectoration disappeared within 20 days. And the bone break was healed within 30 days.

Fractures in General

"An Understanding of the Orthopedic Axiom 'In Treating the Bones, First Treat the Flesh' " by Pan Zhong-heng, *Zhong Yi Za Zhi (The Journal of Traditional Chinese Medicine)*, #12, 1992, p. 54; CC

Over the course of long term clinical practice in orthopedics, Mr. He has summarized the axiom of, "In treating the bone, first treat the flesh," as the single major therapeutic principle among the abundance of theories in Chinese medical orthopedics. This essay is based upon an understanding of two aspects of the theory, "In treating the bone, first treat the flesh." The first takes the perspective of the mechanisms involved in bone injury. Given the application of an external force, when the damage first occurs, the flesh will be damaged prior to the bone, and, moreover, this will be a serious condition.

In this article, the term flesh generally refers to the vessels and sinews as well as the flesh itself. The *Nei Jing (Inner Classic)* says: "The bone is the mainstay, the vessels are the battlements, the sinews are the superstructure, and the flesh is the [exterior] wall." It also states, "The gathering of the vessels binds the bones and promotes flexibility of the joints." (These statements) explain the interrelationship between the bones and the flesh and that, in clinical treatment, one must pay great attention to treating the flesh.

Secondly, strength (*i.e.*, a tissue's breaking point when under greatest stress) and integrity (*i.e.*, a tissue's resistance to deformation) are of primary importance from the perspectives of both biomechanics and the mechanical properties the bone and flesh. Based upon our clinical experience, the strength and integrity of the flesh is much lower than that of the bone, and, when a load is applied to both, the degree to which the flesh sustains damage and destruction is much greater than that of the bone. Because of this, in treating the early stages of bone fractures, one must pay particular attention to damage to the flesh, and in treating the bone, one should in actuality treat the flesh first.

207

Acute Lumbar Sprain

"Semen Sinapis Albae (*Bai Jie Zi*) in the Treatment of Acute Lumbar Strain" by Sun Qian-lin, *Zhe Jiang Zhong Yi Za Zhi (The Zhejiang Journal of Traditional Chinese Medicine)*, #4, 1993, p. 185; CC

Semen Sinapis Albae (*Bai Jie Zi*) has a pungent taste and a warm nature. It functions to warm the lungs and eliminate phlegm, disinhibit the qi and scatter nodulation. The *Ben Cao Gang Mu (Great Outline of Materia Medica)* states that it:

> ...disinhibits the qi and phlegm, eliminates cold and warms the middle, dissipates swelling and arrests pain. It treats dyspnea and cough and pain in the sinews and bones of the lumbar joints.

Based upon its folk usage, the author acquired an empirical prescription employing Mustard Seed in the treatment of lumbar sprain. He tried this in clinic, using it repeatedly, and time and again he achieved a good result. The Mustard Seed is fried until yellow and powdered and then administered with yellow (*i.e.*, rice) wine. If the patient cannot drink alcohol, it may be administered in boiling water. Five grams are administered twice daily. In general a cure is achieved within 1-3 days.

Case history: Male, 28 years old, clothing worker. Two days previously he had moved something in an incautious manner. This caused severe pain and soreness in his lumbar region and limited range of motion. Lumbar flexion and squatting elicited intense soreness and pain. Forward bending was limited to 75 degrees and there was obvious pressure pain bilateral to the fourth lumbar vertebra. He had self-administered *Yunnan Bai Yao* (Yunnan White Medicine) and applied *She Xiang Zhui Feng Gao* (Musk Expel Wind Plaster) but to no avail. Five grams of Semen Sinapis Albae was administered twice with yellow wine. After 1 day's administration, the sensation of s'oreness and pain had diminished slightly and he was able to bend forward. Following 3 days of medication, the lumbar pain had disappeared completely and the range of motion returned to normal.

Ge Gen Tang (Pueraria Decoction)

"The Treatment of 20 Cases of Traumatic Injury with *Ge Gen Tang* (Pueraria Decoction) with Additions" by Qiu Wan-xing, *Zhe Jiang Zhong Yi Za Zhi* (The Zhejiang Journal of Traditional Chinese Medicine), #12, 1993, p. 548; CC

In this clinical study, *Ge Gen Tang* was used to treat 20 cases of traumatic injury characterized by damage to the sinew vessels. Thirteen of the participants were male and 7 were female, and they ranged in age from 13 to 50 years old. The course of illness ranged from 2 to 13 days. All of the cases had experienced a trauma or sprain. Eight of the participants had upper extremity injuries, 9 had lower extremity injuries, and 4 had injuries located in the lumbar region. The joints were most often affected. All had already been treated with Western medications or Chinese medical blood-quickening, stasis-transforming medicinals, but these had produced negligible result.

The basic prescription contained: Radix Peurariae Lobatae (*Ge Gen*), 30g, Herba Ephedrae (*Ma Huang*), 9g, Ramulus Cinnamomi (*Gui Zhi*) 10g, Fructus Forsythiae Suspensae (*Lian Qiao*), 10g, fresh Rhizoma Zingiberis (*Sheng Jiang*), 3 slices, mix-fried Radix Glycyrrhizae (*Zhi Gan Cao*), 6g, Radix Albus Paeoniae Lactiflorae (*Bai Shao*) 15g, and Fructus Zizyphi Jujube (*Da Zao*), 12 pieces.

If the injury was located in the upper extremity, then Rhizoma Curcumae Longae (*Jiang Huang*) and Ramulus Mori (*Sang Zhi*) were added. If the injury was located in the lower extremity or the lumbar

209

region, then Radix Achyranthis Bidentatae (*Niu Xi*) was added. If there was severe pain, swelling, and distension, then Rhizoma Cyperi Rotundi (*Xiang Fu*), Gummum Olibani (*Ru Xiang*), and Myrrha (*Mo Yao*) were added. One *ji* was administered in 2 doses daily. In addition, 100g of Radix Puerariae Lobatae (*Ge Gen*) were decocted in water and applied to the affected area as a hot soak.

Of the 20 cases studied, 6 cases achieved a complete cure following administration of 3 *ji* of the prescription. Fourteen cases were cured following administration of 4-6 *ji* of the prescription.

According to the author, traumatic injury is characterized by damage to the sinew vessels producing qi and blood stasis and inhibition of the channels and connecting vessels. This manifests as swelling and distension, soreness and pain, and limited range of motion. Treatment is indicated to soothe and emolliate the sinew vessels, quicken the blood and arrest pain. *Ge Gen Tang*'s capacity for resolving the muscles and soothing the sinews is very much in keeping with these goals. Pueraria is sweet, pungent, and cool. Used in large doses, it resolves the muscles and soothes and emolliates the sinew vessels. Ephedra is pungent and warm. The *Ben Cao (Materia Medica)* states that it functions to "crack patterns of hardness and accumulation." Further, because of its strength in warming, promoting free flow, and dissipating, it is used to warm and unblock the blood vessels, quicken the blood and unblock the connecting vessels, and to dispel stasis and arrest pain. Its qi and flavor are light and clear. Therefore, it courses and unblocks the muscles and skin on the exterior and resolves accumulations of phlegm and congelations of blood on the interior. Thus, it is a useful medicinal for transforming stasis. Ephedra does have a relatively strong diaphoretic effect. However, when used in the treatment of this pattern, it typically does not produce diaphoresis or any other obvious side effects.

Cinnamon is acrid and warm and unblocks the yang. It assists Ephedra in promoting the free flow and circulation of qi and blood. Peony is sour and assists Pueraria in emolliating the sinews, relaxing tension, and arresting pain as well as mediating the excessively acrid and dissipating properties of Cinnamon and Ephedra. The qi of Forsythia is aromatic and its taste is bitter and pungent. Its is ascending, floating, diffusing, and dissipating functions vigorously course the qi and blood. It treats congelation of blood and accumulation of qi in the 12 channels. Moreover, Forsythia regulates and soothes the pathways, allowing it to guide the other medicinals to the illness. Ginger and Red Dates harmonize the constructive and defensive. *An mo* massage, in conjunction with the application of the prescription as a hot soak, promotes the circulation of blood in the injured area and enhances the therapeutic effect.

Zhen Jiu Tui Na
Acupuncture/Moxibustion & Medical Massage _____

Acupuncture

Hiccup

"Two Case Histories of the Acupuncture Treatment of Hiccup" by Pan Xian-ping, *Si Chuan Zhong Yi (Sichuan Traditional Chinese Medicine)*, #1, 1993, p. 53; BF

This article describes the treatment of two cases of hiccup treated by needling *Tai Chong* (Liv 3) and *Nei Guan* (Per 6).

Case 1. Huang X X, male, 39 years old, Oct. 15, 1990

The patient had had an argument with his neighbor and this had given rise to hiccuping. The hiccuping had lasted for 3 days. He had tried Western medical treatment but without success. He presented with chest oppression, epigastric glomus, pulling pain in his chest and diaphragm when he hiccuped, continuous hiccuping without cessation which had affected his intake of food, tidal fever, night sweats, vexatious heat in his five centers or hearts, insomnia, excessive dreaming, lack of strength in his low back and knees, heart vexation, a red tongue with scant, yellow coating, and a wiry, fine, rapid pulse. His TCM pattern diagnosis was liver depression not soothed, liver and kidney yin vacuity, and *chong qi* stirring (*i.e.*, surging) against the diaphragm.

Nei Guan (Per 6) and *Tai Chong* (Liv 3) were needled bilaterally. Strong stimulation was applied to the needles until the hiccuping stopped. The needles were then retained for another 15 minutes before withdrawing them. The patient was then completely cured and there was no relapse.

Case 2. Liao X X, male, 28 years old, Jan. 10, 1992

The patient habitually had chronic, mild gastritis. This was then followed by an outbreak of bronchitis. For this, the patient had taken various Western medicines after which he developed hiccups. His hiccups came one after the other without stopping. These caused repletion and distention. The nape of his neck was tense, tight, and painful, and there was glomus and distention of his chest and diaphragm. The bitterness (of his suffering) was unspeakable. He had tried various traditional Chinese medicines without result. One treatment as above affected a complete cure.

According to the author, hiccups are primarily due to counterflow qi surging up against the diaphragm. In general, this is due to loss of balance of the qi mechanism of the viscera and bowels. In particular, the liver governs coursing and discharge and it balances and keeps uninhibited the qi mechanism. Further, its channels and vessels traverse the two lateral costal regions (the word *xie* also includes the hypochondrium) and pass through the diaphragm to enter the abdomen. *Tai Chong* (Liv 3) is the source point of the foot *jue yin* liver channel. It is a place where the transportation and flow of the source qi can be affected. Needling *Tai Chong* has the power to course the liver and regulate the qi, level the *chong* and descend counterflow. This is based on the principle of needling below for a disease located above. *Nei Guan* (Per 6) is the *luo* or connecting vessel point of the hand *jue yin* pericardium channel. It connects with the hand *shao yang* triple heater and opens the *yin qiao mai*. It also unites with the foot *yang ming* stomach channel. Therefore, needling *Nei Guan* is capable of opening and descending counterflow qi in several channels. It also

214

balances and harmonizes the qi mechanism of the viscera and bowels. In general, it is able to rectify the qi and descend counterflow, while in particular, it loosens the chest and disinhibits the diaphragm.

Cervical Pain

"The Use of Acupuncture and Moxibustion on the *Jia Ji* Points as the Primary Therapy in the Treatment of 70 Cases of Cervical Nerve Root Pain" by Du Ming-fang & Wang Wei-hong, *Shan Dong Zhong Yi Xue Yuan Xue Bao (The Journal of the Shandong College of Traditional Chinese Medicine)*, #1, 1993, p. 24-5; CC

The authors applied acupuncture and moxibustion to the *Jia Ji* points as the primary therapy in the treatment of 70 cases of cervical nerve root pain between the years of 1986 and 1991. Twenty-five of the participants in this study were male and 45 were female. They ranged in age from 27-65 years old. The duration of their illness ranged from 2 months to 15 years. Fifty-two of the participants had experienced symptoms for from 2 months to 3 years, 11 of the participants had experienced symptoms from 4-5 years, and 7 participants had experienced symptoms for more than 6 years.

The primary points selected were the *Jia Ji* points on both sides lateral to the affected area. *Jian Zhong Shu* (SI 15), *Jian Yu* (LI 15), *Jian Zhen* (SI 9), *Qu Chi* (LI 11), *Wai Guan* (TH 5), *Hou Xi* (SI 3), and *San Jian* (LI 3) were also selected on the affected side. Two of the above points were selected for each treatment, and these ancillary points were rotated with each treatment. One and a half to 2.5 *cun*, filiform needles were routinely sterilized.

The primary points were needled obliquely, while the ancillary points were needled with a perpendicular insertion employing a lifting and

215

thrusting, twisting and shaking manipulation with even supplementation, even draining technique. Once the qi had been obtained, electro-
acupuncture was applied with a G6805-II machine producing a
continuous wave form for 45 minutes. Moxibustion was applied to the
Jia Ji points and *Kun Lun* (Bl 60) such that the skin became red.
Therapy was administered daily and 10 treatments was considered 1
course of therapy. There was a rest period of 3 days before beginning
the second course of treatment, and participants were evaluated for
therapeutic effect after 3 courses of treatment.

Complete cure was defined as the disappearance of symptoms with
radiological findings showing slight enlargement of the intervertebral
spaces, recovery of normal activity, and no recurrence of symptoms
6 months later. Marked effect was defined as the fundamental
disappearance of symptoms, the ability to generally function, and the
ability to sleep at night. Positive changes were defined as slight
improvement in symptoms but a recurrence of fatigue and an
exacerbation of symptoms when exposed to wind, cold, or dampness.
No result was defined as a lack of any improvement in symptoms or
constitution. Based on these criteria, 35 cases (50%) achieved a
complete cure, 23 (32.8%) cases achieved a marked effect, 10 cases
(14.3%) achieved some positive changes, and 2 cases (2.9%) reported
no result. The overall amelioration rate was 97.1%.

Case history: Female, 65 year old. The patient had experienced
stubborn neck pain, dizziness, and vertigo for 5 years. This was
accompanied by soreness and numbness in the upper limbs that had
become worse in the last year. She had been taking muscle relaxants
and anti-inflammatory medications through a local hospital for 2
months, but her condition was gradually worsening. She was first seen
by the author on August 20, 1991. The patient appeared to be
suffering, she had a faded yellow facial complexion, and her lips were
dull and pale. Her tongue was pale, the sides had small petechiae, and
her pulse was deep and rough. Physical examination revealed that
there was obvious pressure pain bilateral to the 2nd-6th cervical

vertebrae. Contraction produced numbness in both of the upper extremities, although it was particularly pronounced on the right side. With the head in a supine position and the neck flexed, the brachialis plexus traction test was positive. Radiological examination revealed varying degrees of osteophytic formation at the anterior margin of 3rd-6th cervical vertebrae, narrowing and degeneration the 5-6th intervertebral spaces, and narrowing of the vertebral foramen.

The conclusion was that the patient suffered from cervical vertebrae disease with degeneration of the intervertebral discs. The Chinese medical pattern discrimination was insufficiency of liver and kidneys, depletion of qi and blood, and a loss of nourishment within the sinew vessels. Treatment was administered as outlined above. With acupuncture and moxibustion, the patient was able to sleep. Following 3 courses of therapy, she was completely cured and, on a follow-up visit, reported no relapses.

Cervical vertebrae disease may have many etiologies, including external trauma, extreme exhaustion, and the contraction of wind, cold, and damp pathogens. 1) Acute trauma or obvious external injury is quite rare. Most often the patient is not even aware of the trauma. Cervical trauma tends to occur in young people, but, after middle age, osteophytic development is the most common etiology. 2) Chronic wear and abrasion may consist of hanging one's head while working. This will definitely cause laxity in the ligaments and joint capsule, leading to vertebral subluxation and creating joint malpositioning. 3) The etiology of intervertebral disc degeneration is universally internal in nature. 4) Congenital factors may be present.

The medicine of our country (*i.e.*, TCM) understands cervical vertebrae disease as being related to kidney vacuity and blood vacuity. External causes include, wind, cold and dampness. The *Nei Jing (Inner Classic)* says: "Wind cold and dampness are the three miscellaneous qi and these combine to produce *bi*." Acupuncture and moxibustion at the *Jia Ji* points provide direct stimulation to the local area. The midline of the spine and the regions lateral to the spine must be discriminated as to whether the governing vessel or the urinary bladder channel is involved, since disease in either channel may result in stiffness and pain in the neck. The (chapter in the) *Ling Shu (Spiritual Axis)*, "Miscellaneous Disease", states: "In the case of neck pain character- ized by inability to bend or lift the head, prick the foot *tai yang*, while if one cannot turn (one's head), prick the hand *tai yang*." Therefore, the point *Kun Lun* (Bl 60) on the foot *tai yang* channel is combined (with the *Jia Ji* points).

Jian Zhong Shu (SI 15), *Jian Zhen* (SI 9), and *Hou Xi* (SI 3) are located on the hand *tai yang* small intestine channel. *Hou Xi* adjunc- tively unblocks the governing vessel. *San Jian* (LI 3) functions to course the channels and benefit the joints and is an empirical point in the treatment neck pain. *Jian Yu* (LI 15) and *Qu Chi* (LI 11) function to unblock the connecting vessels, benefit the joints (along the large intestine channel), and treat numbness. *Wai Guan* (TH 5) courses the channels and quickens the connecting vessels. It primarily treats impaired flexion and extension of the arm and elbow and numbness, soreness, and pain in the hands and fingers.

The combination of the primary points and the adjunctive points are employed with the intention that if governing and the *shao yang* vessels flow freely, if the channels and connecting vessels are warmed and flow freely, if the sinews are soothed and the blood is quickened, and if the qi dynamic is regulated, then there will be no pain.

Shoulder Pain

"The Acupuncture Treatment of 86 Cases of Periarthritis of the Shoulder" by Zhou Qu-zhi, *Shang Hai Zhen Jiu Za Zhi (The Shanghai Journal of Acupuncture & Moxibus- tion)*, #1, 1992 p. 25; CC

In this clinical study, the author needled the point *Ling Xia* in the treatment of 86 cases of periarthritis of the shoulder. This point is located in a depression two *cun* below *Yang Ling Quan* (GB 34) and was tender upon palpation in the patients treated. *Ling Xia* was needled on the side of the shoulder pain or bilaterally if the pain was bilateral. A lifting and thrusting needle technique was employed. The needles were retained for a duration of 5 minutes once the qi was obtained. Patients were then instructed to rotate the affected joint through a wide range of movements. Each treatment lasted 30 minutes and was performed once daily. Ten treatments constituted a single course of treatment. *An mo* (*i.e.*, massage) therapy was performed concurrently with the acupuncture.

According to the author, *Ling Xia* is on the gallbladder channel which runs through the shoulder. This point courses and promotes the free flow of channel qi. Once qi is obtained, a forceful technique must be applied in order to circulate the qi and, therefore, maximize the analgesic effect on the shoulder. When combined with local *an mo* massage treatment, this therapy promotes the flow of qi and blood locally. It is effective whether or not electricity is used (to stimulate the needle). It is the author's opinion that the combination of *Ling Xia* and *an mo* shortens the course of therapy for the treatment of this condition.

Chest & Flank Pain

"The Treatment of 65 Cases of Chest & Flank Pain with Acupuncture" by Huang Jin-quan & Lin Jie-li, *Zhe Jiang Zhong Yi Za Zhi (The Zhejiang Journal of Traditional Chinese Medicine)*, #12, 1992, p. 548; BF

This article describes the treatment of 65 cases of chest and lateral costal pain with acupuncture. They begin with a case history.

Lin X X, male, 27 years old

The patient was tense, agitated, and easily angered. He said that lack of happy resolution of certain family matters had resulted in his feeling aching and needlelike piercing pain in both sides of his chest and lateral costal regions. His signs and symptoms included a red face, chest oppression, torpid intake, a red tongue with thick, yellow coating, and a wiry pulse. Based on these signs and symptoms, it was appropriate to balance and regulate the qi mechanism, open the channels, and quicken the connecting vessels. The points chosen were *Nei Guan* (Per 6) and *Yang Ling Quan* (GB 34). They were first needled to obtain the qi. Then, every 5 minutes, the needles were moved once (*i.e.*, manipulated) with draining technique. The needles were retained 30 minutes. After needling once, the pain was diminished. After needling 3 times, the pain was completely eliminated.

Sixty-five cases of chest and lateral costal pain were treated in the same way. Of these, 50 cases of aching and pain were due to liver qi depression and binding. The remaining 15 cases were due to injury damage (*sun shang*). Of the 65 cases, 50 had their pain eliminated and 12 their pain reduced. Three experienced no result. This yielded a 95.3% amelioration rate.

One-sided Sweating of the Head

"The Treatment of One-sided Sweating of the Head with Acupuncture" by Zhang Li-xin, *Zhe Jiang Zhong Yi Za Zhi (The Zhejiang Journal of Traditional Chinese Medicine)*, #12, 1992, p. 548; BF

This clinical audit describes the acupuncture treatment of 8 cases of sweating on one side of the head and face. Zhang begins by remarking that, in modern Western medicine, such one-sided sweating is regarded as a functional nervous disorder. According to TCM theory, it is associated with lack of consolidation of the defensive qi. This allows the fluids and humors to be discharged outside.

Among the 8 cases treated by Zhang, all were males. Their ages ranged from 21-49 years of age, and the duration of their condition had lasted from as short as 1/2 year to as long as 8 years. They were all treated by needling *Yi Feng* (TH 17) and *Qu Chi* (LI 11) with 28 gauge, 2 *cun* needles. These were inserted to a depth of from 1-1.5 *cun*. Every 5 minutes the needles were moved (*i.e.*, manipulated) and they were retained for a total of 30 minutes. The patients were treated 1 time per day. All cases recovered completely. One case recovered after 1 treatment; 2 cases after 2 treatments; 4 cases after 3 treatments, and 1 case after 5 treatments.

Inability to Ejaculate

"The Treatment of 46 Cases of Inability to Ejaculate By Electro-acupuncture" by He Xin-zhu, *Shan Xi Zhong Yi (Shanxi Traditional Chinese Medicine)*, #6, 1992, p. 39; BF

This clinical audit describes the treatment of 46 cases of inability to ejaculate by electro-acupuncture. The ages of the 46 men ranged from 19-38 years old. The duration of their disease ranged from 1-13 years. Forty-four of the patients suffered from primary onset inability to ejaculate, while 2 suffered from secondary onset inability to ejaculate.

The main points used were divided into two groups. Group 1 consisted of *Shen Ting* (GV 24), *Bai Hui* (GV 20), *Qi Hai* (CV 6), *Guan Yuan* (CV 4), *Zhong Ji* (CV 3), *Yang Ling Quan* (GB 34), and *Tai Chong* (Liv 3). Group 2 consisted of *Da Zhui* (GV 14), *Shen Shu* (Bl 23), *Ci Liao* (Bl 32), and *San Yin Jiao* (Sp 6). Supplemental points consisted of *Shui Dao* (St 28), *Gui Lai* (St 29), and *Hui Yin* (CV 1). Electrodes were attached to either *Guan Yuan* or *Qi Hai* and *Zhong Ji* or *Shen Shu* and *Ci Liao* depending upon which group of points were selected. The two main groups of points were alternated each treatment. Electric stimulation was given via the WQ-10C machine at 60 cycles per minute. Needles were left in place from 24-30 minutes per treatment. One treatment was given per day and 10 treatments constituted one complete course of therapy. None of the patients was treated for more than 3 such courses of therapy.

Cure meant that the patient was able to ejaculate and, in some cases, was able to father a child. Lack of cure meant that after 1 month of treatment, the patient was still not able to ejaculate. Of the 42 patients suffering from primary onset inability to ejaculate, 39 or 92.9% were cured and 3 or 7.1% were not cured. Of the 2 patients with secondary onset inability to ejaculate, 1 was cured and 1 was not. And, of the 2 patients with counterflow ejaculation (into their bladders), both were cured. This resulted in a 91.3% cure rate with an 8.7% failure.

He Xin-zhu notes that, according to TCM theory, failure to ejaculate is mostly categorized as liver qi not coursing with obstruction and stagnation in the channels and connecting vessels. Therefore, the principles for treating this condition in the majority of men are to course the liver, rectify the qi, and open the channels and connecting vessels.

Dysmenorrhea

"Hand Technique & the Treatment of Dysmenorrhea with Acupuncture" by Zhong Ya & Zhang Shou-qun, *Zhe Jiang Zhong Yi Za Zhi (The Zhejiang Journal of Traditional Chinese Medicine)*, #2, 1993, p. 79; BF

This is a report on a comparative study of two acupuncture protocols for the treatment of painful menstruation or dysmenorrhea. Seventy-six women were treated with a combination of acupuncture using the technique known as "setting the mountain on fire" (*shao shan huo*) and moxibustion. Another control group of 40 women received acupuncture with even supplementation/even drainage method. The women in this study presented with aching and pain in their abdomens at the onset or arrival of the menses accompanied by chilled extremities, perspiration, a pale, white facial complexion, nausea, vomiting, etc. Zhong and Zhang primarily attribute these symptoms to cold and dampness damaging the lower burner, settling in the *bao gong*, causing congelation of the menstrual blood.

The 76 women in the warming cold treatment group were needled at *San Yin Jiao* (Sp 6) and *Shui Dao* (St 28) with setting the mountain on fire method. This consists of inserting the needle beneath the skin and manipulating it at each of the three layers, superficial, medium, and deep. Then the needle is withdrawn up to the surface in one quick movement. Traditionally, this technique is believed to lead the warm *wei yang* or defensive yang qi from the superficial level to warm the *ying* or constructive qi within. The needles were withdrawn when the patient felt a warm sensation extend to and reach the area of the disease. Treatment was given approximately every day. In addition, *Guan Yuan* (CV 4) and *Zhong Ji* (CV 3) were moxaed for 20 minutes each day. The 40 women in what Zhong and Zhang refer to as the control group were needled with even supplementation/even drainage at *San Yin Jiao* (Sp 6), *Zu San Li* (St 36), *Guan Yuan* (CV 4), and *Qi Hai* (CV 6). In this case, needles were retained for 30 minutes and treatment was given once per day.

Of the 76 women treated, 28 were between 16-20 years of age, 22 between 21-25, 18 between 26-30, and 8 were over 30 years of age. The shortest disease course was 3 months and the longest was 2 years. Fifty-two women were unmarried and 24 were married. Of the 40 women treated in the other group, 14 were between 16-20, 12 between 21-25, 9 between 26-30, and 5 were over 30 years old. The range of duration of their dysmenorrhea was the same as the other group, from 3 months to 2 years. Twenty-six of these women were unmarried and 14 married. Thirty-one women among the 76 had their dysmenorrhea eliminated, 34 markedly improved, 9 somewhat improved, and 2 experienced no result. This yielded a 85.52% amelioration rate in the women treated by warming cold. Whereas, 13 of the 40 women experienced complete cure, 15 marked improvement, 4 fair improvement, and 8 go no result for a total amelioration rate of only 70%.

"The Analgesic Effect of Acupuncture on Endometriosis Patients" by Ni Sheng-ju, *Shang Hai Zhen Jiu Za Zhi (The Shanghai Journal of Acupuncture & Moxibustion)*, #1, 1992, p. 16; CC

This article describes the treatment of pain due to endometriosis with acupuncture. In this study, there were 54 cases treated, 8 of whom had never been pregnant and 46 of whom had been pregnant. Four cases were in the 21-25 year old age group, 7 cases in the 26-30 age group, 24 cases in the 31-35 age group, 15 cases in the 36-40 age group, and 4 cases in the 41-45 age group. All the participants had been diagnosed with endometriosis and suffered from symptoms such as increasingly painful dysmenorrhea, irregular menstruation, infertility and dyspareunia.

In the Chinese medical treatment of endometriosis, treatment principles for prescriptions include: 1) warming the menses and unblocking the connecting vessels in order to transform stasis; 2) dissipating and resolving to dissipate bondage and transform stasis; 3) rectifying the qi and cracking stasis to dissipate bondage; 4) warming the menses and supplementing the kidneys to transform stasis; and 5) transforming phlegm and softening hardness to transform stasis.

The patients in this study had been treated with Chinese herbal medicine but had not experienced a positive analgesic effect from this therapy. They were then treated with acupuncture and moxibustion with 92.6% effectiveness.

Body points used consisted: *Zhong Ji* (CV 3), *Guan Yuan* (CV 4), *Qi Hai* (CV 6), and *San Yin Jiao* (Sp 6). These were each needled 1 time per week using lifting and thrusting technique with even supplementing and even draining methods. The needles were retained for a duration of 20 minutes and, after 10 minutes, they were manipulated with lifting and thrusting technique so as to elicit soreness, distension, and a sensation of diffusing numbness. Ear points used consisted of Ovary, Sympathetic, and Endocrine points. Each of these had a needle embedded in them 1-2 days premenstrually or during menstruation or one piece of Semen Vaccariae Segetalis (*Wang Bu Liu Xing*) was tapped over each point. The patient was instructed to press these points at least 10 times daily. During each of these sessions, they were instructed to press on the points 10-15 times so as to elicit a bearable degree of soreness and pain. Moxibustion was applied to *Xian Bai* (Liv 1), *Yin Ling Quan* (Sp 9), and *Di Ji* (Sp 8). One or 2 points were selected and moxaed for a duration of 5-10 minutes. In cases of chilly pain in the lower abdomen, moxibustion was applied simultaneously with the needles. Two to 3 sessions with body needles and 1 session with ear needles constituted 1 course of therapy. Three courses of therapy were the statistical target.

Over a duration of 1-3 courses of treatment, 7.4% (4 cases) achieved a complete cure. This was defined as an overall disappearance of abdominal pain and cessation of dysmenorrhea for a duration of at least 6 months or the patient became pregnant. Over a duration of 1-3 courses of treatment, 53.7% (29 cases) achieved a marked therapeutic effect. This was defined as a clear diminishment of overall abdominal pain and a discontinuation of the use of analgesics. Over a duration of 1-3 courses of treatment, 31.5% (17 cases) achieved some therapeutic effect. This was defined as a decrease in abdominal pain, dysmenor-rhea, and the need for analgesics. And, over a duration of 1-3 courses of treatment, 7.4% (4 cases) achieved no therapeutic effect.

Menopausal Syndrome

"31 Cases of Menopausal Syndrome Treated by Auriculo-therapy" by Yang Qing-fang, *Yun Nan Zhong Yi Za Zhi (The Yunnan Journal of Traditional Chinese Medicine)*, #5, 1993, p. 27-8; BF

In this clinical audit, 31 women between the ages of 45-50 years old were treated for menopausal syndrome with auriculotherapy. These women suffered from menstrual irregularity, heavy or scant bleeding, episodic sweating, heart palpitations, vexation and agitation, dizziness, tinnitus, and, if severe, emotional depression, unsociability, paranoia, and wild thoughts, insomnia, excessive dreams, easy excitability, etc. Of the 31 cases, 3 were between 42-45 years of age, 19 between 46-50, 8 between 51-55, and 1 was 62 years old. The main points used in this treatment method were: Heart, Liver, Kidney, Subcortex, Sympathetic (Nerve), Internal Secretion, and Uterus.

If there was heart vexation, insomnia, and excessive sweating, then Spirit Gate, Brain, Lungs, and Small Intestine were added. If there was intestinal and stomach discomfort or constipation, Spleen, Stomach, Large Intestine, and Small Intestine were added. If menstru-ation was chaotic, Uterus, and Ovaries were added. If there was obesity, Spleen, Spirit Gate, Flesh Drop (*i.e.*, Weight Loss), Mouth, Large Intestine, and Ridge Mound were added. If there were heart palpitations and chest oppression, Sympathetic (Nerve), Small Intestine, and Spirit Gate were added. And if there was high blood pressure, Spirit Gate and Lowering Pressure Groove were added. These points were stimulated by taping Semen Vaccariae Segetalis

(*Wang Bu Liu Xing*) onto each point in the ear bilaterally. Each time, 2-3 different points were selected. These were left in place for 3 days and the patient was instructed to press them 3-5 times per day. Ten treatments (*i.e.*, 30 days) constituted 1 course of treatment.

Marked results were defined as complete disappearance of the (above) conditions or their obvious diminishment and, after ceasing treatment for 1 whole month, no recurrence. Good results were defined as partial disappearance of the (above) conditions or a turn for the better. And no result was defined as no obvious improvement in the (above) conditions or a turn for the better but a return of symptoms 1 week after discontinuing treatment. Of the 31 cases so treated, 11 experienced marked results, 17 good results, and 3 no results for a total amelioration rate of 87%.

Neurodermatitis

"The Treatment of Neurodermatitis with Auriculo-acupuncture" by Wang Mei-hua & Yue Dong-shan, *Bei Jing Zhong Yi (Beijing Traditional Chinese Medicine)*, #6, 1992, p. 42; BF

This clinical audit discusses these two doctors' research on the auriculo-acupuncture treatment of neurodermatitis. Wang and Yue treated 69 cases of neurodermatitis using the following auricular points. Main points: *Fei* (Lungs), *Pi Zhi Xia* (Lower Skin), and *San Jiao* (Triple Heater). If there was severe itching, *Shen Men* (Spirit Gate) was added. If heat was severe, *Er Jian* (Ear Apex) was added. If the emotions were not easy, *Xin* (Heart) was added. If the disease had lasted a long time without being cured, *Zhen* (Pillow) was added. If heat and itching were extremely severe, *Er Jian* (Ear Apex) was bled. Ears were first disinfected. Then 0.5 *cun* filiform needles were inserted on one side only in 4-6 points per time. The needles were only retained a short period of time and were manipulated once during that period. One treatment was given per day with 10 treatments constituting 1 course of therapy. If no result was obtained after 5 treatments, treatment was stopped without doing the entire course.

Cure consisted of elimination of the dermatitis with no recurrence within 3 months. Improvement consisted of elimination of dermatitis but recurrence within 3 months. No result meant that there was no change after the treatment from before in the dermatitis. Of the 69 cases treated, 10 were cured after 1 course of therapy, 49 after 2-3 courses. Thus the total number cured was 59 or 85.51%. Another 9 (13.04%) experienced improvement and only 1 (1.45%) failed to register any improvement. Therefore the total amelioration rate was 98.55%.

Pediatric Enuresis

"The Acupuncture Treatment of 62 Cases of Pediatric Bed-wetting" by Bao Bei-yi, *Zhong Yi Za Zhi (The Journal of Traditional Chinese Medicine)*, #1, 1993, p. 26; BF

This report describes the acupuncture treatment of 62 cases of pediatric enuresis or bed-wetting. There were 37 boys and 25 girls among this group. They ranged in age from 5 years to 17 years old with most of the children falling between 6-10 years of age. The shortest duration of this condition had lasted half a year and the longest 12 years. Thirty-five children wet their beds 1-2 times each night, 17 children wet their beds 3-4 times each night, and 10 children wet their bed 1 time every several nights.

Treatment consisted of needling *Tong Li* (Ht 5) and *Da Zhong* (Ki 4). *Tong Li* was needled to a depth of 3 *fen* and manipulated with draining technique. *Da Zhong* was also inserted to a depth of 3 *fen* and manipulated with supplementation technique. The needles were retained for 10-15 minutes. In addition, *Guan Yuan* (CV 4) was moxaed for 3-5 minutes. One treatment was given per day and 6 treatments constituted 1 course of therapy. Thirty-five of the 62 cases were completely cured after 1 course of therapy; another 21 were markedly improved; and 4 were somewhat improved. Two cases failed to experience any result. The total amelioration rate in this research was 96.8%.

Pediatric Night-crying

"The Treatment of 13 Cases of Pediatric Night-crying" by Liu Bai-sheng, *Jiang Su Zhong Yi (Jiangsu Traditional Chinese Medicine)*, #2, 1993, p. 30; BF

This clinical audit describes the treatment of 13 cases of pediatric night-crying. (The translator's opinion is that this is the traditional Chinese name for what is known as pediatric colic in English.) There were 7 boys and 6 girls in this group ranging in age from 2-10 months of age. The duration of this disease was mostly 2-3 months. The points needled consisted of *Si Feng* (M-UE-9) and *Da Ling* (Per 7). Both points were treated bilaterally. The *Si Feng* points were needled with a triangular needle to a depth of 1 *fen*. Then the points were squeezed manually until a yellowish white fluid or a drop of blood were expressed. *Da Ling* was needled with a fine needle with even supplementation, even drainage hand technique for 1 minute. The needles were not retained. One treatment was given per day and the night crying completely disappeared in all 13 children after 3 treatments. Lui says that needling *Si Feng* and *Da Ling* resolves heat and eliminates vexation, tranquilizes the heart and calms the spirit, opens the intestines and the hundred vessels, regulates and harmonizes the viscera and bowels.

Tourette's Syndrome

"A Report on the Treatment of 156 Cases of Tourette's Syndrome with Acupuncture" by Yi Lian-chong *et al.*, *Zhong Yi Za Zhi (The Journal of Traditional Chinese Medicine)*, #7, 1993, p. 423-4; BF

This clinical audit discusses the specifically acupuncture treatment of 156 cases of pediatric Tourette's Syndrome in 1991. One hundred two of these cases were boys and 54 were girls. Thus the ratio of boys to girls was 1.5:1. One hundred fourteen cases were between 6-10 years of age, and 42 were between 11-15. the course of disease ranged from as short as 6 days to as long as 1 year. Seventy-eight cases had already been treated with modern Western medicine and 36 cases had received Chinese medicinals and acupuncture. During their previous treatment, 144 cases had received electroencephalography with 84 showing some abnormality. All the children had been x-rayed, with 6 showing some abnormality there. In addition, 84 had received CAT scans, with 6 abnormalities found.

According to the authors, sufferers of this syndrome can be divided into two patterns: 1) *yang ming* heat accumulation pattern and 2) sea of marrow insufficiency pattern. The signs and symptoms of the *yang ming* heat accumulation pattern are a strong, fat constitution, a moist, red face, the repeated emission of vocal sounds, twitching of the facial region with possible constipation, a red, moist tongue with a thick, slimy, possibly yellow coating, and a flooding, large or slippery, rapid pulse. Based on these signs and symptoms, 66 of the 156 children were categorized as manifesting this pattern. The signs and symptoms of the sea of marrow insufficiency pattern are a weak, emaciated body constitution, and ashen white facial color, less emission of vocal sounds, slow, gentle twitching of the skull and body, clear, disinhibited urination or frequent urination, a pale, fat tongue, and a fine, weak pulse. Based on these symptoms, 90 of the 156 cases were categorized as manifesting this pattern.

The treatment principles for the *yang ming* heat accumulation pattern were to clear and discharge the *yang ming*. This was accomplished by using the lifting and thrusting draining method at *Nei Ting* (St 44), *Qu Chi* (LI 11), and *Pian Li* (LI 6). Sparrow-pecking draining method was used at *Si Bai* (St 2). After obtaining the needle sensation, the needles were not twisted. The treatment principles for the sea of marrow insufficiency pattern were enrich the kidneys, nourish the heart, and regulate the *du* (*mai*). This was accomplished by using the twisting and rotating supplementing method at *Shen Men* (Ht 7) and *Fu Liu* (Ki 7). *Ya Men* (GV 15) was needled to a depth of between 1.5-2 *cun* until an electric sensation was felt in the upper extremities emanating from the needle. And *Lian Quan* (CV 23) was needled using sparrow-pecking method until the area felt distended. One treatment was given per day with the needles retained for 30 minutes. Every 10 minutes, the needles were stimulated 1 time. Two weeks of such treatment equalled 1 course of treatment.

Cure consisted of complete disappearance of the twitching and vocalization with no recurrence of this condition. Control of this condition meant that the twitching was reduced in frequency and intensity and the symptoms were mostly diminished. If there was no obvious improvement in the symptoms after 3 complete courses of treatment, this was defined as no result. Based on these criteria, 114 or 73.1% were cured, 30 or 19.25 were brought under control, and 12 or 7.7% experienced no result. Thus the combined amelioration rate was 92.3%. Eighty-one point eight percent of those categorized as manifesting the *yang ming* heat accumulation pattern were cured as compared to 66.7% of those manifesting the sea of marrow insufficiency pattern being cured.

According to the authors of this report, most convulsive disorders are categorized as liver wind in TCM. However, in the case of this disease which occurs in children, it should not be treated as wind stroke. Heat accumulating in the *yang ming* is due to lack of discipline in food and drink coupled with the child's inherent flourishing yang constitution. Whereas, sea of marrow insufficiency is due to former heaven (*i.e.*, prenatal) insufficiency, *i.e.*, kidney essence deficiency and vacuity. In the former case, accumulated heat in the *yang ming* transforms into fire and engenders wind. In the latter case, essence fails to nourish the ancestral sinews, treasure essence, and act as residence of the source spirit. Thus in the former case, treatment is directed at points on the *yang ming*, while in the latter case, points on the kidney and heart channels and conception and governing vessels are selected.

Moxibustion

Suppurative Moxibustion

"The Clinical Use of Suppurative Moxibustion" by Li Mingzhi, *Shang Hai Zhen Jiu Za Zhi (The Shanghai Journal of Acupuncture & Moxibustion)*, #3, 1992, p. 33-4; CC

Suppurative moxibustion is an ancient moxibustion technique, the administration of which is quite painful and leaves a permanent scar. Under normal conditions, patients are generally unwilling to submit to this technique. However, since suppurative moxibustion at local acupoints enhances and prolongs the positive (therapeutic) stimulus within the body, it can, therefore, have an unusual effect on (the treatment of) recalcitrant diseases. Following administration of suppurative moxibustion, one may often observe the immediate resolution of lingering illness. The *Zi Sheng Jing (The Classic of Nourishing Life)* states that, "All moxa should must produce a sore in order for the patient to recover." As a result of this, it would seem that suppurative moxibustion has a distinctive therapeutic effect. The following selection of case histories illustrates its clinical value.

1. Herniation of a lumbar disc

Tian, a 35 year old male carpenter, was first diagnosed on August 20, 1987. He complained of left-sided lumbar and leg pain that had lasted for half a year. The pain radiated from his lumbar region along his urinary bladder channel (with pain) shooting into his foot such that he was unable to walk. It was also difficult for him to turn over.

Examination revealed a severely laterally rotated torso and lateral prominence (of the bulging disc) on the affected side. The patient had a positive straight leg raise test (*i.e.*, a Cram test. This is accomplished by the examiner raising the straight leg. This will cause pain. The knee is then slightly flexed while the thigh remains in the same position. This causes the pain to disappear. Next, thumb or finger pressure is then applied to the popliteal area to reestablish the painful radicular symptoms.) He also had a positive bowstring test and a positive Kernig test (*i.e.*, Kernig-Brudzinski test. In order to perform this test, the patient lies supine with their hands cupped behind their head. They are then instructed to flex their head to their chest. Next, the extended leg is actively raised by flexing the hip. The test is positive if pain is felt.) There was (also) pressure pain in the L4-5 intervertebral space, and percussion produced a shooting pain. And there was obvious pressure pain at *Cheng Fu* (Bl 38) and *Wei Zhong* (Bl 40). Radiology reported herniation of the lumbar disc at the L4-5 level.

The patient had undergone a combination of massage, acupuncture, and Chinese herbal therapies and, over the past 2 months, his symptoms had improved somewhat in that he was now able to walk approximately 30 meters. Nevertheless, the lateral rotation remained severe, lumbar flexion was still difficult, and the straight leg raise test remained positive. (Conventional) moxibustion was added to the therapy for 1 month but produced no major progress.

Finally, suppurative moxibustion was administered. The selection of points included: *A Shi* points (*i.e.*, trigger points lateral to the spine), *Cheng Fu* (Bl 38, left), *Wei Zhong* (Bl 40, left). A major moxa burn was induced with the radius of the base area being raised approximately 1cm. This was accomplished with 4 cones of moxa to produce a second degree burn. Self-composed *Jiu Cang Gao* (Moxa Sore Ointment) was applied topically to the moxa burn. After 4 days, the moxa sore opened and suppurated for a period of 34 days. On the 15th day of suppuration, the patient returned to our clinic for a follow up visit. The patient's back had become perfectly straight and he was so overjoyed that he was nearly delirious. After 1 month, the straight leg raise test was negative, the bowstring test was negative, the Kernig test was negative, and he walked normally. In a follow-up visit three years later, he reported no recurrence of the symptoms.

2. Heel pain

Jiang, a 86 year old male, was first examined in July of 1988. He had been experiencing left heel pain for the past 6 months and this made walking difficult. The radiology report indicated heel spurs. He had been to a public hospital and had undergone both Chinese and Western therapies. The application of plasters, anti-inflammatories, and medicinals, such as *Gu Ci Pian* (Anti-osteophyte Pills) and *Fu Fang Ruan Gu Su Pian* (Softening the Bone Compound) had been ineffective. Examination revealed obvious pressure pain on the medial aspect of the left heel and pressure pain 1cm below the acupoint *Zhao Hai* (Ki 6). First the point, *Zhao Hai Xia* (Below Shining Sea, an experiential point) was needled with a filiform needle on the left side, followed by (the needling of) reactive points on the palm of the right hand. Therapy was administered 1 time per day for 10 consecutive treatments. Although the symptoms diminished somewhat, walking continued to produce heel pain.

Five days later, the patient returned for treatment. Suppurative moxibustion was applied directly to *A Shi* points (*i.e.*, the painful points on the bottom of the heel). Since the skin on the heel was thickly calloused, a fire needle was employed. In other words, the point was pricked 4 times instead of using 4 cones of moxa. And _Jiu Cang Gao_ was applied topically to the needle hole. In 3 days, the needle hole suppurated. After 2 weeks, the sore had scabbed over and the heel pain had completely disappeared. Re-examination 2 years later revealed no recurrence of symptoms.

3. Dysmenorrhea

Xu, a 40 year old female, was first examined on April 21, 1989. Menarche had occurred at 14 years of age and she had married at age 20. After 1 year of marriage, she gave birth to a single child. At age 22, an inadvertent fall brought on midcycle menstruation. After this, her menstruation became so painful that she was bedridden. She had since suffered from dysmenorrhea for 18 years and treatment at both Western and Chinese hospitals had proved futile. Gynecological examination revealed a soft abdomen without masses or appendages. There was no cervical dysplasia, no uterine tumors, nor was there any vaginal or uterine inflammation. Her facial complexion was slightly yellow, she had an aversion to cold and liked warmth, and she had a small volume of menstruate which contained clots. Her tongue was pale purple with a thin, white coating and her pulse was fine and wiry. The pattern discrimination was cold in the sea of blood with stasis obstructing the uterus. Therefore, therapy was aimed at warming the menses and quickening the blood.

Chinese medicinal therapy consisted of _Si Wu Tang_ (Four Materials Decoction) with the additions of Ramulus Cinnamomi (_Gui Zhi_), Radix Praeparatus Aconiti Carmichaeli (_Fu Zi_), Rhizoma Corydalis Yanhusuo (_Yuan Hu_), and Rhizoma Cyperi Rotundi (_Xiang Fu_). Acupuncture and moxibustion were administered to _Guan Yuan_ (CV 4, warm needle), _Guan Yuan Shu_ (Bl 26, warm needle), _He Gu_ (LI 4), and _San Yin Jiao_ (Sp 6). Prior to each cycle, 5 _ji_ were administered and acupuncture and moxibustion were administered 5 times. With continuous therapy over the course of 3 menstrual cycles, the dysmenorrhea had diminished slightly. However, when acupuncture and herbal therapy were discontinued over the course of the 4th menstrual cycle, abdominal pain increased again in intensity.

Thus, suppurative moxibustion was indicated. An *A Shi* point was selected — a trigger point 1 *cun* above *Guan Yuan* (CV 4). Over the next 32 days, the moxa sore suppurated. Eight months later, she made a special visit to report that, following the suppurative moxibustion, she had experienced a complete cure of her dysmenorrhea within 2 menstrual cycles. She had experienced no abdominal pain over the subsequent 6 months. On a follow-up call a year later, she reported that the ailment had not returned.

The above cases were all recalcitrant (to prior treatment). However, with appropriate use of suppurative moxibustion technique, one treatment affected a cure and the long-term therapeutic effects were excellent.

Tui Na

Upper Abdominal Pain

"385 Cases Utilizing Measures for Coursing the Channels & Rectifying the Qi in the Treatment of Localized Upper Abdominal Pain" by Zhang Zhen-xing, *Zhong Guo Zhong Xi Yi Jie He Za Zhi (The Chinese Journal of Integrated Chinese-Western Medicine)*, #2, 1992, p. 124; BF

In this study, musk plasters were used in conjunction with *an mo* finger pressure in the treatment of upper abdominal pain. A *Hu Gu She Xiang Gao* (Tiger Bone Musk Plaster, also known as Jaku

Kokotsu in the US) or a *Ru Xiang Zhui Feng Gao* (Tracing Wind Plaster) was applied to a sore area in the gastric region. The patient then massaged the specific points with his middle finger for a duration of 5 minutes, 3 times daily so that a strong needling sensation was elicited. Points normally chosen included *a shi* points, *Shang Wan* (CV 13), *Zhong Wan* (CV 12), *Liang Men* (St 23), *Tian Shu* (St 25), *Nei Guan* (Per 6), and *Zu San Li* (St 36). One course of therapy lasted 3 days.

The duration of illness ranged from 10 minutes to 30 years, and the age of the patient ranged from age 10 to over 40. Two hundred fifty-six cases were acute, and 120 were chronic. The range of illnesses with which these patients had been diagnosed included duodenal ulcer, enteritis, cholecystitis, cholelithiasis, ascariasis, and gastric ulcer. Therapy was judged effective if there was complete disappearance of the pain.

This technique enhances the therapeutic effect of other modalities. It is simple and uncomplicated. The massage may be applied by physicians or patients alike and is safe. It may be used alone, when medication has proven to be ineffective, or it may be combined with medication. As such, its use merits popularization.

Torticollis

"Tui Na Combined with the Topical Application of Medicinal Paste in the Treatment of Stiff Neck (literally, dropped pillow)" by Qiu Jing-chuan, *Shang Hai Zhong Yi Yao Za Zhi (The Shanghai Journal of Traditional Chinese Medicine 7 Medicinals)*, #5, 1992, p. 17; BF

The patients in this study ranged in age from adolescents to middle-aged. The duration of their illness ranged from 1-3 days. The following techniques were applied with the patient sitting:

1. *An Rou*/Press & knead technique at *Feng Chi* (GB 20), *Tian Zong* (SI 11), *Jian Zhong Shu* (SI 15)

2. Massage of the neck and spinal areas combined with lateral stretching and twisting movements

3. *Na Fa*/Grasping technique at *Feng Chi* (GB 20), *Feng Fu* (GV 16), and up and down 3-5 times from the flesh of the neck at *Jian Jing* (GB 21)

4. *Yao Ban Fa*/Shaking and pulling technique on either side of the cervical vertebrae, once at each vertebrae

5. Based on a discrimination of patterns of either wind, cold, stasis, or taxation and whether sleeping movements aggravate the situation, either *Zhi Shang San, Ding Gui San,* or *Qi Li San* (available in prepared form) were given. (In addition,) *Jie Jing Zhi Tong Ding* (Resolve the Channels, Stop Pain Tincture) was dripped onto these medicinal powders to moisten them into a paste. This was applied to the cervical region for a duration of 24 hours. It was then removed for 4-6 hours after which time they were administered again.

Eight cases achieved a complete recovery; 6 cases achieved disappearance of cervical pain, although a sensation of stiffness remained; and one case achieved no therapeutic effect.

Miscellaneous Articles _____

Chuan Xiong Cha Tiao San

"New Uses for *Chuan Xiong Cha Tiao San* (Ligusticum & Tea Regulating Powder)" by Miao Hou-qing, *Zhe Jiang Zhong Yi Za Zhi (The Zhejiang Journal of Traditional Chinese Medicine)*, #4, 1993, p. 184; CC

In this article, the author discusses several new uses of this famous formula. It is most usually employed in the treatment of headaches, nasal congestions, and illnesses of the head and face. The formula itself is composed of: Rhizoma Ligustici Wallichi (*Chuan Xiong*), Herba Seu Flos Schizonepetae Tenuifoliae (*Jing Jie*), Radix Ledebouriellae Sesloidis (*Fang Feng*), Herba Cum Radice Asari Sieboldi (*Xi Xin*), Radix Angelicae (*Bai Zhi*), Herba Menthae (*Bo He*), Radix Glycyrrhizae (*Gan Cao*), and Radix Et Rhizoma Notopterygii (*Qiang Huo*)

Urticaria

Case history: Male, 52 years old. The patient had suffered from generalized itching and welts for 4 days. This was accompanied by abdominal pain, diarrhea, vomiting, and a simultaneous sense of chills and fever. His temperature was between 37.8-38.5°C. He had taken Western medicine and his abdominal pain and vomiting had diminished somewhat, but his skin symptoms remained unbearable. The welts varied in size, were pale red in color, and were worse on the abdomen and inside of the legs. The patient was agitated and had aversion to wind and cold. A scratch test was positive. His pulse was wiry and tongue was pale and white. His TCM diagnosis was external contraction of wind cold with failure of harmonious circulation of qi and blood. The treatment principles were to eliminate wind, dissipate cold, resolve the exterior, circulate the qi, and quicken the blood. He took 1 *ji* of this formula per day, once in the morning and once at night. After 3 *ji*, he was much improved. With 6 *ji*, his condition was consolidated.

The disease mechanism of this condition primarily relates to wind. As our predecessors have said, "To treat wind, first treat the blood; if the blood circulates, then wind will be extinguished of its own accord." However, in treating the blood, one must also circulate the qi, since "the qi is the master of the blood" and "if the qi circulates, the blood will circulate." Ligusticum is a qi within the blood medicinal. Therefore, it is used to nourish and quicken the blood and circulate the qi. It regulates the blood within the entire body. Schizonepeta, Ledebouriella, Angelica, Mint, and Asarum course wind, dissipate cold, and arrest itching. Licorice harmonizes these other medicinals. While Tea's bitter, cold nature moderates the warming nature of the other medicinals.

Rheumatoid Arthritis

Case history: Female, 32 years old. The patient had suffered from recurrent generalized muscle soreness for 2 years which was worse with changes in the weather. Anti-inflammatories and analgesics were ineffective. On examination, the patient presented with contracted extremities which were not red and swollen but were cold. She had difficulty walking on her left lower leg. In addition, she had aversion to wind and cold. The pain lacked a fixed location. Her pulse was wiry and tense, and her tongue was pale with a white coating. Her TCM diagnosis was wind cold *bi zheng*. The treatment principles were to eliminate wind, dissipate cold, quicken the blood, and arrest pain. After 3 *ji*, all her symptoms diminished and she could walk on her left leg. After 15 *ji* she was cured.

Wind cold may enter the body, lodging in the muscles and sinews. In that case, circulation of qi and blood will be impaired resulting in pain. Schizonepeta, Ledebouriella, Asarum, and Notopterygium all are pungent and warm and disperse cold and eliminate wind. Mint also strongly eliminates wind but when combined with Tea, it mediates the hot effect of the other medicinals. While Ligusticum circulates the qi and quickens the blood, eliminates wind and arrests pain.

Premenstrual headache

Case history: Female, 39 years old. The patient had been suffering from premenstrual headache for more than 20 years. These headaches were cyclic in nature. She would develop a mild headache 2 days prior to her period which would gradually increase in intensity until the onset of her menstruation, at which time it would disappear. The pain was frontal and supraorbital and she would often use heat resolving analgesics. She generally took 1-2 aspirin per day to relieve the pain. However, in the past 2 years, even 3 aspirin were ineffective. (The consulting physician) happened to examine her 2 days prior to her period when the headache was present and she was already in severe pain. Her pulse was wiry and her tongue was pale with a thin, white coat. The physician administered *Chuan Xiong Cha Tiao San*, 1 *ji* decocted in water and administered in two doses, morning and evening. Administration of Western medication was suspended. After administration of a second *ji*, the headache was significantly diminished. This protocol was used for the 3 days prior to the next 5 periods. She took a total of 17 *ji*, and the premenstrual headaches disappeared altogether. Her medication was then discontinued and 3 months later she reported no recurrence of symptoms.

Premenstrual headache is seldom (*sic*) seen in clinical practice. In this case, the illness was of a long-standing nature, manifesting prior to each menses. According to the theory, "At the beginning, an illness lies within the channels, while a chronic illness enters the blood", the

241

correct treatment is normally to both nourish and quicken the blood. The use of medicinals for eliminating wind would seem to run contrary to normal reason. However, *Chuan Xiong Cha Tiao San*, which primarily eliminates wind and secondarily quickens the blood, achieved a cure (in this case). This is because medicinals for dispelling wind are not exclusively indicated for short term illnesses in which there an externally contracted headache due to a wind pathogens. This class of medicinals may also be used in some long-term illnesses when combined with medicinals for blood vacuity and blood stasis.

Wan Dai Tang

"New Uses for *Wan Dai Tang* (Arresting Vaginal Discharge Decoction)" by Qian Sheng, *Zhong Yi Za Zhi (The Journal of Traditional Chinese Medicine)*, #9, 1993, p. 550; CC

Wan Dai Tang consists of stir-fried Rhizoma Atractylodis Macroce-phelae (*Chao Bai Zhu*), stir-fried Dioscoreae Oppositae (*Chao Shan Yao*), Radix Panacis Ginseng (*Ren Shen*), stir-fried Herba Seu Flos Schizonepetae Tenuifoliae (*Chao Jing Jie*), stir-fried Radix Albus Paeoniae Lactiflorae (*Chao Bai Shao*), Rhizoma Atractylodes (*Cang Zhu*), stir-fried Semen Plantaginis (*Chao Che Qian Zi*), Pericarpium Citri Reticulatae (*Chen Pi*), Radix Bupleuri (*Chai Hu*), and Radix Glycyrrhizae (*Gan Cao*). It is quite effective for gynecological conditions. The authors have expanded its scope of application based upon its functions of supplementing the middle and strengthening the spleen, transforming dampness and arresting leukorrhea. What follow are a number of representative cases.

Chronic diarrhea.

Case history: A 47 year old male was first examined on October 12, 1988. He had been suffering postprandial diarrhea for 1 year. Western medical examination revealed nothing unusual and repeated Western medical therapies were ineffective. If he consumed even the slightest bit of oily or greasy food, the diarrhea would return. When he was examined, he reported having 3-5 bowel movements per day which were watery in nature or watery and contained undigested grain. He had no abdominal pain and little appetite. He was slightly emaciated and lethargic. His tongue was pale and there were tooth marks on the sides. The tongue coating was moist and white, and his pulse was vacuous and lacked strength. The diagnosis was diarrhea due to a vacuity of stomach and spleen, water dampness assaulting the spleen, and a descent of damp turbidity.

For this case, it was appropriate to supplement the middle transform dampness, and arrest diarrhea. Therefore, *Wan Dai Tang* was administered with modifications. It consisted of: stir-fried Rhizoma Atractylodis Macrocephelae (*Chao Bai Zhu*), 30g, stir-fried Radix Dioscoreae Oppositae (*Chao Shan Yao*), 30g, Radix Codonopsis Pilosulae (*Dang Shen*) 15g, stir-fried Herba Seu Flos Schizonepetae Tenuifoliae (*Chao Jing Jie*), 4g, stir-fried Radix Albus Paeoniae Lactiflorae (*Chao Bai Shao*), Rhizoma Atractylodis (*Cang Zhu*), 12g, stir-fried Semen Plantaginis (*Chao Che Qian Zi*), 12g, Pericarpium Citri Reticulatae (*Chen Pi*), 3g, Radix Bupleuri (*Chai Hu*), 4g, stir-fried Fructus Crataegi (*Chao Shan Zha*), 15g, and Terra Flava Usta (*Cao Xin Tu*), 50g (precooked). After administration of 3 *ji* of this prescription, the patient's stools became sticky and diminished in frequency to 2-3 times per day. His appetite also returned. He continued taking another 5 *ji* of the same prescription and his stools became formed and further diminished in frequency to twice a day. One year later, the patient reported no recurrence of symptoms.

Somnolence

Case history: A 35 year old female was first examined on May 6, 1990. Two months previous, she had developed a generalized fever and body ache after being soaked in a drenching rain. This was treated successfully. However, she became somnolent. When examined, she reported that she was experiencing fatigue and somnolence, heaviness in her head and body, diminished appetite, a bland taste in her mouth and lack of thirst, soft, pasty stools, clear, long urination, and a clear, thin vaginal discharge. Her tongue was pale and had a thin, white coat, while her pulse was soggy and moderate. The diagnosis was a vacuity of stomach and spleen and dampness assaulting spleen yang.

Treatment to supplement the middle and fortify the spleen, transform dampness and unblock the yang was, therefore, indicated. She was administered *Wan Dai Tang* with modifications. This consisted of: stir-fried Rhizoma Atractylodis Macrocephelae (*Chao Bai Zhu*), 30g, stir-fried Radix Dioscoreae Oppositae (*Chao Shan Yao*), 30g, Radix Codonopsis Pilosulae (*Dang Shen*), 15g, Rhizoma Atractylodes (*Cang Zhu*), 12g, stir-fried Semen Plantaginis (*Chao Che Qian Zi*), 12g, Pericarpium Citri Reticulatae (*Chen Pi*), 6g, Radix Bupleuri (*Chai Hu*), 6g, Ramulus Cinnamomi (*Gui Zhi*), 8g, Radix Ledebouriellae Sesloidis (*Fang Feng*), 6g, Sclerotium Poriae Cocos (*Fu Ling*), 6g, and Rhizoma Acori Graminei (*Shi Chang Pu*), 6g. Three *ji* of this prescription was administered in decoction and all of her symptoms diminished. With administration of 3 more *ji*, all of her symptoms disappeared completely and did not return.

Wan Dai Tang was first developed for the treatment of abnormal vaginal discharge by Fu Qing-zhu. The prescription contains doses of as much as 30g of Atractylodes and Dioscorea which focus on supplementing the middle and fortifying the spleen. It can be very effective in the treatment of patterns characterized by middle warmer depletions when modified accordingly. In the first case, Terra Flava Usta was added to the basic prescription to warm the middle, astringe the intestines, and arrest diarrhea. Crataegus was added to supplement the spleen, transform stagnation, and arrest diarrhea, and the sour Fructus Schizandrae (*Wu Wei Zi*) was also added to arrest diarrhea. All of these additions addressed the branch symptom. In the second case, Cinnamon was added to unblock the yang and transform water. Ledebouriella was added to dispel wind and overcome dampness. Poria was added to supplement the spleen and percolate dampness. And Acorus was added to open the stomach and arouse the spirit.

Slimy Yellow Tongue Coating

"A New Perspective on Slimy Yellow Tongue Coating" by Ma Min-fu & Xu Lian-fang, *Zhe Jiang Zhong Yi Za Zhi (The Zhejiang Journal of Traditional Chinese Medicine)*, #12, 1993, p. 567; CC

A slimy, yellow tongue coating is a manifestation of a damp heat pathogens which are usually appropriately treated via the methods of clearing heat and disinhibiting damp, clearing heat and drying damp, and the use of aromatic medicinals for transforming turbidity. However, in clinical practice, these treatment methods frequently yield an unsatisfactory result. In clinical practice, when diagnosing and treating a patient with a slimy, yellow tongue coating, the authors often use medicinals for warming and transforming damp cold, and this approach often produces an immediate effect. The disease mechanism is as follows:

Dampness is a yin pathogen and, once it stagnates, it is not easy to expel. Long-standing depression of a damp pathogen will transform to heat, which, in turn, will express itself in a slimy, yellow tongue coating. Regardless of how yellow the tongue coating is or how slimy or thick it might be, there must be a significant or at least a slight white tongue coating present either in the middle or at the base of the tongue. This is the key piece in the discrimination of patterns. If the patient has this tongue coating, then the root of illness is cold and damp, while the branch illness is damp heat. Therefore, the use of methods to warm and transform cold damp are indicated. This removes the fire from beneath the cauldron (*i.e.*, treats the situation at its source), treating the root and thus eliminating the illness. If instead one uses methods for clearing heat and drying dampness, clearing heat and disinhibiting dampness, or employs aromatic medicinals for transforming turbidity, this is like trying to stop water from boiling by scooping it out of the pot and then pouring it back in. It will be difficult to eliminate the pathogen.

Index of Author's Names _____

247

O, P, Q

R, S

T

W

X

Y

Z

D

D & C 71
Da Ling 229
Da Zhong 228
Da Zhui 221
depression, emotional 126
Di Ji 225
diabetes mellitus 194
diaphragm, distention and oppression of the chest and 33
diarrhea, acute 28
diarrhea, chronic 28, 242
diarrhea, long-term ceaseless 25
diarrhea with pain relieved after diarrhea 26
dizziness 33, 35, 40, 45, 53, 72, 78-79, 84, 87-88, 95, 97, 124, 126, 128-129, 142, 145-146, 153, 159, 200, 216, 226
dreaming, excessive 1, 35, 53, 54, 64, 78, 87, 146, 189, 218, 226
drinks, desire for warm 10
dryness syndrome, senile 4
dysentery 28
dysmenorrhea 65, 99, 101, 103, 120, 150, 222-226, 235, 236
dyspnea and rough respiration 10

E

ears, ringing in the 20, 72, 142, 153
ectopic pregnancy 130-134, 136
eczema 153, 194
edema, climacteric 146
ejaculate, inability to 221, 222
ejaculation, premature 156, 159
emaciated physical form 154
emotional affairs, lack of ease in 89
emotional anxiety 165

emotional depression 126, 226
emotional lability 1, 32, 96
emotions not normal 38
endometriosis 73, 75, 78, 99, 101, 103, 105-108, 125, 149, 224
enema, retention 25, 27, 107, 159, 160
eructation, sour 22
eruptions, polymorphous sunlight 190, 192
excitability, easy 226
extremities, chilled 11, 223
extremities, edematous swelling of the lower 138
extremities, numbness in four 59
extremities, weakness of 88
extremity injuries, lower 209

F

face, red 10, 220, 230
facial color, ashen, stagnant 22
facial color, ashen white 129, 230
facial complexion, sallow, white 11
facial complexion, white 11, 12, 223
facial lustre, diminished 84
fatigue and somnolence 244
fatigue, exhaustion and 53, 54
fatigue, spiritual 21, 22, 84
Fei Shu 13-14, 166, 167
Feng Chi 238
Feng Fu 238
fever 56-58, 159, 168, 169, 178, 182, 213, 239, 243
fever, tidal 213
flus, recurrent 1
fright 56-58, 155
Fu Liu 231
Fu Qing-zhu 244

G

G6805-II machine 216
Gao Huang 13
gastric fullness 169
gastric *pi* 11
genitalia, edematous swelling of external 138
GB 20 238
GB 21 238
GB 34 219-221
Ge Shu 13
glomus, epigastric 213
Great Outline of Materia Medica 208
Guan Yuan 221-223, 225, 229, 235, 236
Guan Yuan Shu 235
Gui Lai 221
GV 14 221
GV 15 231
GV 16 238
GV 20 221
GV 24 221

H

hair tends to be fine and yellowish, sparse 165
hands and feet, heat in the center of 34, 172
He Gu 235
headaches, bilateral 19
headache, frontal 19
headache, one-sided 19
headache, premenstrual 241
headache, vascular 19
head and body, heaviness in 244
head, one-sided sweating of 220
heart vexation 53, 54, 172, 189, 200, 213, 226

heat *bi* 52
heel pain 45, 46, 49, 234, 235
hematuria 159
hemoptysis, perimenstrual 78
herpes zoster 176-178, 180, 181, 183-185, 187
hiccup 213
Hou Xi 215, 218
Ht 5 228
Ht 7 231
Hui Yin 221
hunger, easy 68

I

impotence 153-155, 157, 159
infection, upper respiratory 167
infertility 157, 224
inhalation, difficult 12
Inner Classic 70, 207, 217
insomnia 1, 19, 20, 35, 40, 53, 54, 59, 145, 213, 226
intake, diminished 11
torpid intake 27, 40, 118, 141, 142, 179, 220
intercourse, pain with 102
intermenstrual phase 114, 117
internal medicine 1, 29
itching 4, 13, 42, 64, 86, 139, 175, 176, 178, 182, 191, 193, 198, 200, 227, 239, 240

J

Jia Ji points 215-218
Jian Jing 238
Jian Yu 215, 218
Jian Zhen 215, 218
Jian Zhong Shu 215, 218, 238
Jing Yue Quan Shu 28, 63

V

vagina, irregular bleeding from 131
vaginal discharge, abnormal with offensive odor 125
vaginal discharge, abnormal, white 111
vaginal discharge, clear, thin 244
vaginal discharge, excessive 64, 111
vaginal discharge, excessive, pasty white 87
vaginal itch 64, 86, 139
vaginal tract, excessive bleeding from 82
Valium 53
vertex, pain at the 19
vertigo 40, 64, 72, 95, 97, 153, 200, 216
vexation and agitation 42, 64, 74, 126, 145, 226
vexatious heat in the five centers 56, 58, 116, 142, 213
vocal sounds, repeated emission of 230
voice, hoarse 4
voice, weak, forceless 11
vomiting 33, 78, 90, 135, 168, 169, 223, 239
vomiting of phlegmy saliva 90

W, X

Wai Guan 215, 218
Wai Ke Zheng Zong 91
warts, facial flat 197
weak body 17, 165
weeping with grief, easy 144
Wei Zhong 233, 234
wheezing 6-14
wind, intestinal 28
Women's Department Secrets 127
Wu Kun 71

x-ray 18, 46
Xian Bai 225

Y

Ya Men 231
Yang Ling Quan 219-221
Yi Lin Gao Cuo 58, 60
Yin Ling Quan 225
yin ju 147

Z

Zhang Jing-yue 28, 67, 75
Zhao Hai 234
Zhao Hai Xia 234
Zheng Zhi Hui Bu 9
Zhong Ji 221-223, 225
Zhu Bing Yuan Hou Lun 77
Zi Sheng Jing 232
Zu San Li 223, 237

Formula Index

263

SOMETHING OLD, SOMETHING NEW; Essays on the TCM Description of Western Herbs, Pharmaceuticals, Vitamins & Minerals by Bob Flaws ISBN 0-936185-21-X $19.95

A NEW AMERICAN ACUPUNCTURE: Acupuncture Osteopathy, by Mark Seem, ISBN 0-936185-44-9, $19.95

SCATOLOGY & THE GATE OF LIFE: The Role of the Large Intestine in Immunity, An Integrated Chinese-Western Approach by Bob Flaws ISBN 0-936185-20-1 $12.95

MENOPAUSE, A Second Spring: Making A Smooth Transition with Traditional Chinese Medicine by Honora Lee Wolfe ISBN 0-936185-18-X $14.95

MIGRAINES & TRADITIONAL CHINESE MEDICINE: A Layperson's Guide by Bob Flaws ISBN 0-936185-15-5 $11.95

STICKING TO THE POINT: A Rational Methodology for the Step by Step Administration of an Acupuncture Treatment by Bob Flaws ISBN 0-936185-17-1 $14.95

ENDOMETRIOSIS & INFERTILITY AND TRADITIONAL CHINESE MEDICINE: A Laywoman's Guide by Bob Flaws ISBN 0-936185-14-7 $9.95

THE BREAST CONNECTION: A Laywoman's Guide to the Treatment of Breast Disease by Chinese Medicine by Honora Lee Wolfe ISBN 0-936185-13-9 $8.95

NINE OUNCES: A Nine Part Program For The Prevention of AIDS in HIV Positive Persons by Bob Flaws ISBN 0-936185-12-0 $9.95

THE TREATMENT OF CANCER BY INTEGRATED CHINESE-WESTERN MEDICINE by Zhang Dai-zhao, trans. by Zhang Ting-liang ISBN 0-936185-11-2 $16.95

A HANDBOOK OF TRADITIONAL CHINESE DERMATOLOGY by Liang Jian-hui, trans. by Zhang Ting-liang & Bob Flaws, ISBN 0-936185-07-4 $14.95

A HANDBOOK OF TRADITIONAL CHINESE GYNECOLOGY by Zhejiang College of TCM, trans. by Zhang Ting-liang, ISBN 0-936185-06-6 (2nd edit.) $21.95

PRINCE WEN HUI'S
COOK: Chinese Dietary
Therapy by Bob Flaws &
Honora Lee Wolfe, ISBN 0-
912111-05-4, $12.95 (Published by
Paradigm Press, Brookline, MA)

THE DAO OF
INCREASING LONGEVITY
AND CONSERVING ONE'S
LIFE by Anna Lin & Bob Flaws,
ISBN 0-936185-24-4 $16.95

FIRE IN THE VALLEY:
The TCM Diagnosis and
Treatment of Vaginal
Diseases by Bob Flaws
ISBN 0-936185-25-2 $16.95

HIGHLIGHTS OF
ANCIENT ACUPUNCTURE
PRESCRIPTIONS trans. by
Honora Lee Wolfe & Rose
Crescenz ISBN 0-936185-23-6
$14.95

ARISAL OF THE CLEAR:
A Simple Guide to Healthy
Eating According to
Traditional Chinese Medicine
by Bob Flaws, ISBN #-936185-
27-9 $8.95

CERVICAL DYSPLASIA &
PROSTATE CANCER:
HPV, A Hidden Link? by Bob
Flaws, ISBN 0-936185-19-8
$23.95

PEDIATRIC BRONCHITIS:
ITS CAUSE, DIAGNOSIS &
TREATMENT
ACCORDING TO

TRADITIONAL CHINESE
MEDICINE trans. by Gao Yu-li
and Bob Flaws, ISBN 0-936185-
26-0 $15.95

AIDS & ITS TREATMENT
ACCORDING TO
TRADITIONAL CHINESE
MEDICINE by Huang Bing-
shan, trans. by Fu-Di & Bob
Flaws, ISBN 0-936185-28-7
$24.95

ACUTE ABDOMINAL
SYNDROMES: Their
Diagnosis & Treatment by
Combined Chinese-Western
Medicine by Alon Marcus, ISBN
0-936185-31-7 $16.95

BEFORE COMPLETION:
Essays on the Practice of
TCM by Bob Flaws, ISBN 0-
936185-32-5, $16.95

MY SISTER, THE MOON:
The Diagnosis & Treatment
of Menstrual Diseases by
Traditional Chinese Medicine
by Bob Flaws, ISBN 0-936185-
34-1, $24.95

FU QING-ZHU'S
GYNECOLOGY trans. by
Yang Shou-zhong and Liu Da-
wei, ISBN 0-936185-35-X,
$21.95

FLESHING OUT THE
BONES: The Importance of
Case Histories in Chinese
Medicine by Charles Chace.
ISBN 0-936185-30-9, $18.95

CLASSICAL MOXIBUSTION SKILLS IN CONTEMPORARY CLINICAL PRACTICE by Sung Baek, ISBN 0-936185-16-3 $10.95

MASTER TONG'S ACUPUNCTURE: An Ancient Lineage for Modern Practice, trans. and commentary by Miriam Lee, OMD, ISBN 0-936185-37-6, $19.95

A HANDBOOK OF TCM UROLOGY & MALE SEXUAL DYSFUNCTION by Anna Lin, OMD, ISBN 0-936185-36-8, $16.95

Li Dong-yuan's TREATISE ON THE SPLEEN & STOMACH, A Translation of the *Pi Wei Lun* by Yang Shou-zhong & Li Jian-yong, ISBN 0-936185-41-4, $21.95

PATH OF PREGNANCY, VOL. I, Gestational Disorders by Bob Flaws, ISBN 0-936185-39-2, $16.95

PATH OF PREGNANCY, VOL. II, Postpartum Diseases by Bob Flaws, ISBN 0-936185-42-2, $18.95

How to Have a HEALTHY PREGNANCY, HEALTHY BIRTH with Traditional Chinese Medicine by Honora Lee Wolfe, ISBN 0-936185-40-6, $9.95

MASTER HUA'S CLASSIC OF THE CENTRAL VISCERA by Hua Tuo, translated by Yang Shou-zhong, ISBN 0-936185-43-0, $21.95